DREAM CHAPTER

Design Your Meaningful Retirement

A Collection of Stories

Charlie Baker,
Larry Wofford,
and Craig Bothwell

Copyright © 2022 by Charlie Baker, Larry Wofford, and Craig Bothwell

ISBN 979-8-9854549-0-1
eISBN 979-8-9854549-1-8

Published March 2022

Table of Contents

Preface

A retired partner from a large accounting firm called requesting to meet with me. The next day we sat down to coffee in my small conference room. I asked, "How's retirement life?"

The look in his eyes startled me as much as his words, "Why didn't you prepare me for retirement?"

"What do you mean?" I asked.

He answered, "This is the hardest transition I have ever gone through. I'm confused, angry, and depressed. Retirement is so hard. Why didn't you prepare me?"

Wow. For more than twenty years my specialty as an executive coach at one of the largest accounting firms in the world included preparing people for advancement. I worked with people receiving promotions, preparing them for new responsibilities. I helped people work through difficult assignments to maximize the impact of their time and work.

Preparing people for retirement?

Raised on a ranch, I was not hardwired in my youth to even think about retirement. Ranchers don't retire — they just run fewer cattle. After countless interviews with retirees and those preparing to retire, I arrived at this strong conclusion: retirement is a key transition, perhaps the most important we ever make. Yet despite its importance, most people give little thought or develop a strategy for how to approach the unexpected changes. I heard a financial planner say, "The average person spends more time planning a wedding than planning for retirement."

Significant issues arise for those not financially prepared for retirement. But more often, the regrets we hear center around a lack of planning for meaning and quality of life following retirement. We hear the refrain:

"I woke up retired and wondered what the heck to do with the rest of my life."

This problem stems from assuming retirement opens freedom to play and do all the things not possible under the constraints of a job; however, for most people, play and leisure do not hold the equivalent motivational force of meaningful work. The leisure associated with fun and games provides a certain level of value but does not generate the powerful sense of a worthwhile life.

The drive for fulfillment, living a life of worth and value, continues throughout life. At no point or age does the desire for worth and value disappear. Harry Truman, back home in Missouri after leaving the White House, went for a walk one day with a friend. They passed a man they knew to be 99 years of age who walked slowly, in obvious pain. The friend said, "Who would want to be 100?"

Truman replied, "That guy!"

Having a strong sense of purpose in life leads to improvements in both physical and mental health and enhances the overall quality of life. It may extend life itself.

In plain English, if you find a life purpose, you will probably live both longer and better than someone without a life purpose.

Something deep within each of us enjoys and finds worth in meaningful accomplishments. Exploring possible ways to build purpose, value, and choices in retirement makes life an exhilarating adventure producing a new sense of freedom.

As one retiree said, **"I find myself more interested in discovering who I am and what I can meaningfully do with my life now than at any time since high school or college graduation."**

The privilege of speaking at over 300 funeral and memorial services through the years taught me a lot about life's purpose. I make it a practice to meet with the family and friends of the deceased a day or two before the service, to listen to their thoughts about their loved one. I always ask, "What would you like me to say about him or her?" Not one time out of those hundreds of conversations did I ever hear anyone say, "Be sure to tell them he or she had a net worth of so many dollars, a certain amount of money in the bank, and owned a lot of stuff." Not one time.

Instead, they told me about how the person touched the lives of others. They wanted me to give tribute to the contributions made through their work, communities, places of worship, and families. They focused on the sacrifices made for family, country, or some worthy cause. We tend to think accumulating wealth brings satisfaction and comfort. It does not. Wealth is good and helpful and important, but it does not give meaning to life.

During the retirement transition, you encounter chances to strategize and plan how you will use your time, talents, experiences, and resources to continue to live in a meaningful way. With this kind of plan, you look forward to getting up in the morning and getting on with the day to see how your "meaningful" investments are adding up instead of checking the stock market.

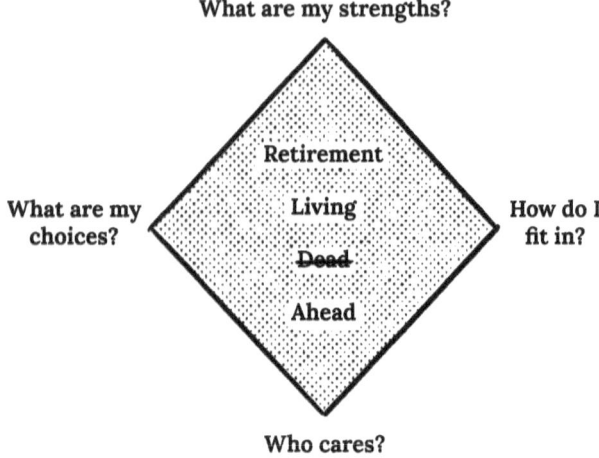

Four key life questions I use in leadership development or crisis management work also apply to retirement planning. These questions prompt healthy thinking and help prepare for the transition to retirement:

1. Who am I with my strengths?

    As we age, we lose some physical strength and certain abilities. Muscles weaken, eyesight dims, and hearing fades. But other areas grow stronger, so play off your strengths, not your weaknesses. Planning how to use your strengths in

10

retirement pays excellent dividends. Everyone offers something to give others when they identify their strengths.

2. Where do I fit in?

Either consciously or subconsciously, all of us desire to fit in. Looking at a puzzle on the table, we search for the pieces to complete the picture. We want to belong. We long to participate in something important and meaningful. We desire acceptance rather than being viewed as an outsider. Focusing our retirement strategy on the places we fit helps us avoid a great deal of unhappiness.

3. Who cares?

This question consists of two parts. The first is how do you care for yourself? And the second is how do you care for others? This requires a constant balancing act, and you need both to experience a fulfilling life. Focusing on only one or the other creates imbalance, burnout, and physical plus emotional stress. Keep both in mind as you make your plans.

4. What are my choices?

    The world proclaims, "You can be anything you want to be", but that is not true. We all have finite physical, mental, and financial resources which may not match what we want them to be. The important thing is to determine what is within your control, what is available, and then how you will decide between the realistic choices in front of you. Stretch yourself to recognize the difference between possible and fantasy. When you make better choices, you find a better life.

This book helps you answer these four key questions. As I began researching and interviewing to prepare and equip myself to coach people on this important life transition of retirement, I also started looking for other coaches with a similar interest. Believing issues of great challenge find the best solutions through a team approach, I joined two other coaches, Craig Bothwell and Larry

Wofford. Both have coached many individuals in different career tracks and life situations. We share similar views on the need for retirement preparation.

Retirement needs conversion from an event to a seamless life transition.

Forming a team allowed us to bring a wider variety of perspectives, experiences, and stories to this book. Our collective experience, tempered with research and study, equips us to bring value to people in or nearing retirement. We encourage you to view retirement more as where you are going than where you have been or where you are. Therefore, we challenge you to continue living with intentionality and focus during retirement.

We guide you in understanding the important difference in long-term satisfaction between leading a life of leisure and leading a leisurely life.[1]

---

[1]   The difference between a life of leisure and a leisurely life is described by Dr. Richard P. Johnson in *The New Retirement*, second edition, Columbus, OH: Career Partners International, LLC, (2019), p 98.

We use techniques in our coaching practice to move you from thinking in terms of feedback to using the concept of *feedforward to fuel continuous improvement.* We think where you are going is far more important than where you have been. These straightforward perspectives help you create a life just as exciting in retirement as when you first entered the workforce. Let's work together to prepare you to live every day in retirement to the fullest.

Our overall goal is to help you continue to become the best possible version of yourself.

This book is presented as journey "episodes". Each episode highlights an actual coaching experience from one of the three authors. The client names in the episodes have been changed in the interest of confidentiality and the stories are not verbatim in the interest of keeping them a workable length. However, these coaching experiences provide insights into common retirement issues. Throughout the book, you will see "I" in the episodes and other places. Don't let the pronoun confuse you as it is used to represent different authors throughout the book.

Discoveries found along the way follow each "journey". After the discoveries, we challenge you to apply the ideas to your own quest for a meaningful retirement. We conclude with a change of pace, a short comment or quotation from a wiser source than us, echoing the heart of each episode. In it, we hope you find a seed thought for planting or a brain spark for igniting future fruitfulness and light.

" *Retirement is a career, not a vacation, and the benefits are awesome!* **"**

CRAIG BOTHWELL

Introduction

Why this Book Is Important to Your Retirement Success

Retirement is Your Unique Dream Chapter

If you think of your life journey as a book, retirement is the "Dream Chapter". It should be the chapter in which you, as the story's hero, map the course to your buried treasure. Retirement is the segment of your life when time becomes plentiful. Perhaps for the first time in your life, you have the freedom to pursue your purpose and follow wherever the winds of your heart lead.

Viewed as part of your life story, retirement seems simple. You've worked all your life and retirement means no more work: a permanent vacation! Your part is to retire and do whatever comes naturally, which ought to result in a meaningful and satisfying retirement. However, our experience with pre-retirees and retirees indicates that like other life transitions, a satisfying retirement is neither inevitable nor easy. Retirement can become a source of joy and engagement, but it can also lead to boredom, loneliness, and despair. Many people do not instinctively know how to retire successfully, even when money and health are not issues.

To understand this, just look at the numbers. Recent research indicates that in a large sample, 48.6% of retirees classify their retirement experience as "very satisfying", the equivalent of "great". Another 40.9% of retirees rate retirement as "moderately satisfying", the equivalent of "okay". The remaining 10.5% rate retirement as "not at all satisfying", the equivalent of "awful". This means that slightly over half of retirees worked 40 or more years, only to experience an okay or awful retirement. There was no significant difference between how men and women rated their retirement satisfaction.[2]

These numbers indicate retirement is not an easy, fool-proof path to life satisfaction. A 50-50 chance of experiencing your Dream Chapter awaits you. And these numbers are *optimistic*! Why? Because this research only assesses life satisfaction at *a single point in time*. Our experience indicates a high percentage of retirees had to learn to adapt to retirement life before they were able to experience high levels of life satisfaction. Even then, highly satisfied retirees must stay committed to sustaining a meaningful and satisfying retirement by constantly adapting.

---

[2] Employee Benefit Research Institute, "Trends in Retirement Satisfaction in the United States: Fewer Having a Great Time," Sudipto Banerjee, April 25, 2016. Accessed at https://www.ebri.ort/content/trends-in-retirement-satisfaction-in-the-united-states-fewer-having-a-great-time-3342 on 11/26/2021.

Retirement Should Be the Dream Chapter of Your Life Story.

You have a lot to contribute to the world, your friends, your family, and yourself. The odds of enjoying a very satisfying retirement should be better than a coin toss. This short book will improve your odds of designing and living a purposeful, mindful, meaningful, satisfying, and sustainable retirement. The few hours or so it takes to read this book and consider the information and questions within it will provide significant returns in retirement success.

This Book Is Not About the Financial Aspects of Retirement

We understand the importance of money in retirement, but we also understand purposeful retirement is more closely related to your mindset than your bank account. We've watched retirees with all levels of financial resources succeed at retirement and struggle with retirement. This book deals with the non-financial aspects of retirement satisfaction. Many good financial advisors and books are available to help you succeed financially. Our focus in this book is on maximizing your chances of successful retirement *life*.

Read and Engage

This book informs. Simply reading it will make you aware of the value of planning for the non-financial aspects of your retirement. Reading *and* engaging with the questions and exercises in the book will produce even greater benefits for you. Thoughtfully answering the questions and completing the exercises will expand your thinking. Conversations with your significant other, family members, and trusted friends will further expand your awareness and thinking. So, please view this book as an active participation project, not just another quick read. By doing so, you can begin to design your unique retirement strategy.

If you have a significant other contemplating retirement or already retired, this book offers challenging questions and exercises for conversations leading to great retirement strategies. The best way to find powerful answers is to ask powerful questions. Better questions lead to better answers. Honestly challenge yourself with the questions. Take *all the time* you need to find your specific and unique answers.

Assess Your Retirement Mindset

You likely have a dominant mindset, a worldview you routinely bring to daily life. Your mindset affects what you see, how you perceive it, and how you react or respond to it. Our experience suggests individuals work from a dominant, or default, mindset, and an additional mindset to which they can easily "flex". For example, the mindset used at work may differ from the mindset used at home. Throughout your life, you have shifted your mindset to match the tasks and relationships at hand. The importance of mindset awareness continues in retirement as you seek to match the right mindset with changing circumstances. Being in your "right mind", whichever mind is best for a given situation, is a valuable life skill. In each episode in this book, attention is given to the impact of mindset.

Our experience indicates that potential retirees and retirees tend to exhibit four general mindsets:

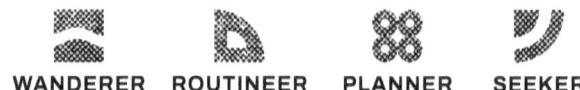

WANDERER   ROUTINEER   PLANNER   SEEKER

Each of these mindsets demonstrates different behavioral tendencies affecting your ability to realize purpose and meaning. You likely display one of these four mindsets as your "home base". The intensity of the primary mindset can vary significantly as, for example, some "planners" are zealous while others are less so. You may flex from your primary mindset as necessary, but your primary mindset generally remains the default.

In just a few minutes you can assess your primary and flex Retirement Mindsets using our 15-question Retirement Mindset Quiz at:

www.dreamchapter.com/survey

As you review your Retirement Mindset results, think about your primary mindset, as well as your flex mindset or mindsets. Throughout the remainder of this book, consider how your mindsets affect your behavioral tendencies in retirement.

THE FOUR RETIREMENT MINDSET PROFILES

To make the Retirement Mindsets more vivid, personal, and useful, consider the details of each of the following mindsets. As you read about each mindset, think about when and how often you exhibit the characteristics of that mindset. Also, consider what you might need to change about yourself to use the mindset effectively.

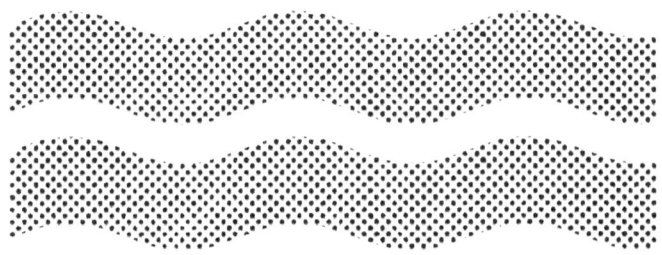

THE WANDERER

"I desire to explore new things in retirement, but I have historically yielded to the expectations of others. My challenge is to decide what I want to do now and then do it."

What Does Retirement Look Like to Wanderers?

At first, retirement appears to be an exciting time because Wanderers have lived a dutiful and structured life to please others in their work and at home. Conforming to the expectations of others drives their decision making, but retirement provides the chance to be more single-minded in what they want to pursue.

Wanderers think, "Now is my time to explore and wander freely for a while. I've earned it and don't want to squander this opportunity."

At the same time, Wanderers will have a challenging time taking control and self-generating activity since they have depended on others for guidance and motivation.

Retirement Danger for Wanderers

Wanderers tend to think about a lot of things they want to start doing, but they also tend to procrastinate. They are mentally imaginative but challenged when it comes to execution.

This drives Wanderers from a state of early optimism to pessimism. With expectations and high hopes, the failure to move forward quickly solidifies their sense of being *stuck*.

The danger is drifting here and there in an unintentional state, wishing to do more interesting things, but not doing them.

What Wanderers Need Most

Wanderers need to learn how to narrow in and select what they desire to explore from their expansive options; then find a way to plan out the actions to start them and keep them on the path.

What holds Wanderers back in retirement is failure to focus, plan, and act when they own total charge of themselves. They need help getting started and staying going.

How Dream Chapter Can Help Wanderers

Our program helps Wanderers be decisive about defining and selecting what they want to do based on their own interests. Then we help plan the steps giving them structure and accountability. We guide them out of wandering and into the discovery of the greatest meaning and purpose in retirement.

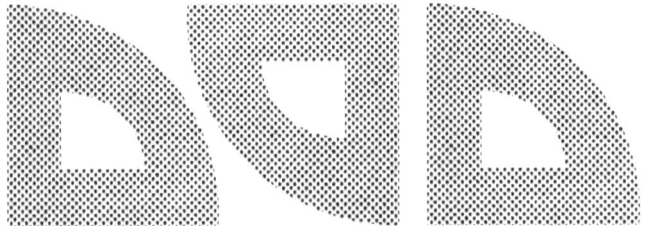

THE ROUTINEER

*"I have enjoyed the same comforting,
purposeful, and predictable routine
for years. Now in retirement, how do
I figure out how to fill this big chunk
of time? I'm worried about finding the
repeatable day-in, day-out activities
not requiring me to think, 'What
am I going to do next?'"*

What Does Retirement Look Like to Routineers?

The great thing about work for Routineers is how easy it is to design their habits and routines. Just like anyone else, they approach retirement with positivity because freedom, at least in the abstract, is exciting.

However, they know themselves well. Routine brings them comfort. It provides a steady purpose not needing to be questioned. It provides a level of busyness and contentment.

Retirement for Routineers becomes the search for a new set of routines providing reliable daily structures of balance and comfort.

The beat goes on for them. They need to find it quickly to replace the rhythm of work routines.

Retirement Dangers for Routineers

Routineers suddenly break from routine at retirement. They feel anxiety and view the hours of extra time daily as a challenge to overcome. Routineers rapidly adopt anything at hand to build a new routine.

The danger is failing to take time to be intentional. Their search requires patience. Their temptation is to jump to the nearest rock rather than seek their most meaningful dream chapter island. Rigidness blocks Routineers from trying new things or spontaneously "going with the flow" when others invite them to join in new activities.

When Routineers create a new set of routines, they may create a difficult rut to leave. Retirement may become depressing and boring. Because routine is everything, it becomes a trap limiting future possibilities.

What Routineers Need Most

Routineers need routine and structure to provide them with meaning and happiness. They need to learn how to add new things into their routine. These don't need to be grandiose bucket lists.

Routineers must be comfortable spending more time in the exploring and planning phase. This is a scary place for them, but with the right guidance and structure, they can learn how to do this and beat the demons of anxiety and boredom.

How Dream Chapter Can Help Routineers

Our program helps Routineers recognize the shocks they will feel in the transition and reassures them that tackling unstructured time is their major challenge.

Instead of trying to turn them into swashbuckling adventurers, our program helps them pause a little longer and look beyond their normal horizons. They will learn how to take small steps. Relaxing their rigid mindset, they find valuable new things to add to their satisfying routines.

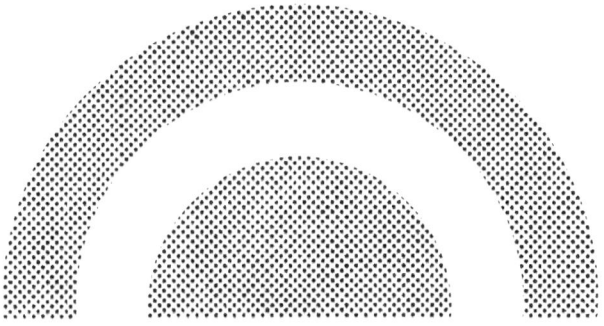

THE SEEKER

"I want to pursue many ideas and opportunities in retirement. I have been effective at accomplishing my goals, but if I'm not intentional about setting priorities and seeing them through, I could end up over-extending my time and resources."

What Does Retirement Look Like to Seekers?

Seekers tend to approach retirement as a new beginning rather than an ending, and they eagerly dive into this next challenge.

Adventurous and willing to try new things, they view their newfound free time as an opportunity to pour themselves into the interests and projects missed in the past. In fact, because of their entrepreneurial mindset and strong sense of purpose, Seekers may take on an entirely new "career" after retirement.

For the Seeker, retirement is anything but a reason to slow down. Wanting to avoid idle time, they may have several new endeavors lined up before they ever step away from their job.

Their fearless drive and eagerness to take on new things make retirement an exciting time. However, Seekers need the right balance and the ability to prioritize their pursuits, or they may end up feeling unfulfilled and overextended.

Retirement Dangers for Seekers

The danger is seeing the blank slate of retirement and trying to fill it with too much. Seekers may underestimate the time and resources required to accomplish their excessive goals. The result is beginning projects with great ambition and purpose only to end up dropping the ball mid-way through to pursue something else.

Lack of accomplishment becomes disheartening for Seekers. They end up exhausted, unfulfilled, and feel like they squandered their retirement on too many meaningless activities.

What Seekers Need Most

Seekers need to learn how to focus on priorities and to direct their time, energy, and resources towards creating a meaningful impact in a few specific areas that matter most to them.

What blocks Seekers is failing to pause, seek advice, and think through the full implications before taking on something new.

How Dream Chapter Can Help Seekers

Our program helps Seekers focus on their priorities and create a plan for what they will (and will not) pursue in retirement. We help Seekers channel their powerful, ambitious energy towards activities creating the greatest sense of fulfillment and purpose in their lives.

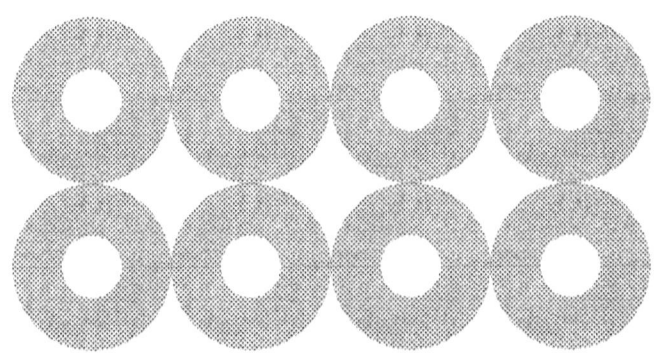

THE PLANNER

"I am financially prepared and have a plan for my retirement. I have been anticipating this transition and realize that it will be an adjustment, but by setting goals and intentionally structuring my time, I feel empowered and in control of my retirement as long as everything goes according to plan."

What Does Retirement Look Like to Planners?

Planners feel ready to take on retirement as long as they've been given adequate time to create a plan and fill their retirement itinerary with trips, activities, and projects for the first few months or even years.

The last thing Planners want is to feel idle or bored, so they take charge of retirement by making plans. They'll leave the office and board a plane for vacation on their last day of work, then have golf plans with friends, pottery classes, or family visits all lined up. Planners may even have a pretty good idea of where they'll be four or five years into retirement.

Having a plan helps this retiree feel in control. Given ample time to prepare, Planners can approach retirement confidently and optimistically. However, if Planners are thrown into retirement unexpectedly, they'll end up feeling completely directionless and unequipped.

Retirement Dangers for Planners

The danger with Planners is the tendency to cram the blank space of retirement with rigid structure. This structure may interfere with enjoying the moment or pivoting to pursue new and more fulfilling opportunities.

Freedom to live in the moment discovering new interests can be one of the greatest joys of retirement, but Planners deny themselves this adventure when they insist on living life according to the plan. The spontaneous getaway or the brand-new, joy-giving hobby are rejected because the plan is set in stone.

What Planners Need Most

Planners need to learn how to keep their plan flexible and embrace the freedom to discover new activities and opportunities. Planners get stuck in the familiar without thinking big enough about the possibilities of action and accomplishment in their retirement. They need help coming up with pursuits for finding fulfillment and openness within new possibilities.

How Dream Chapter Can Help Planners

Our program helps Planners think bigger about their retirement and set growth-oriented goals to stay fulfilled and not just busy. We challenge Planners to leave room in their retirement for intentional spontaneity. We help them identify when it's time to break the plan to pursue something even better.

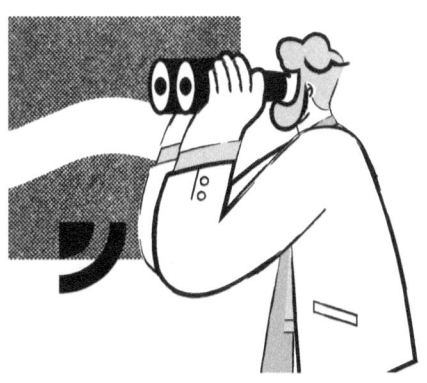

Alex the WANDERER

" *Purpose is feeling like the world needs you as much as you need it, that you have something to contribute and that you still matter.* **"**

MARC FREEDMAN, CEO OF ENCORE.ORG

What can a man four times retired (so far) teach you about purpose in life?

Focus

Our society sends many mixed messages about personal value and how your value gets determined. Beginning in our youth, we receive praise from a parent or teacher for complying with rules and/or outstanding performance of tasks given to us. In school, the best students and/or athletes receive the honors and awards. In the workplace, those who perform with excellence rise through the ranks. (Sometimes the advancements, unsurprisingly, fall on those who married the owner's son or daughter!) Obviously, separating our performance from purpose is difficult. And retirement magnifies this issue.

Society shouts, "Do something to be somebody!" Truth whispers, "You are somebody, now go do something." We are not human doings. We are human beings. Each of us holds an inner treasure of inestimable worth and value. *Learning how to find fulfillment and purpose, especially when in or nearing retirement, is of great value.* If you find nothing to live for, why keep on living? The famous football coach Bear Bryant told reporters through the years, "I'd croak in a month if I quit coaching." And he did. He died 28 days after his final game.

Alex's Journey into Meaning and Purpose

Alex's story differs from other journeys shared in this book. Neither a client, a co-worker, nor a stranger, he coached my football team when I was 12 years old. One day in practice another boy's helmet crashed into my face. My teeth and lower lip went into a bloody rearrangement. Coach Alex provided immediate first aid and encouragement, helping me be brave and calm in the midst of pain. Later in the evening, he called my parents to follow up on my condition and give suggestions to improve the healing process.

I reacted by thinking, "I want to be like him when I grow up." I understood Alex's real aim extended far beyond coaching football. Alex communicated a deep caring for his students, coworkers, friends, and family. Our hometown invented a citizenship award to honor Alex and made his character the standard for future award winners. Even now at the age of 90, his actions of constant care continue.

When we asked Alex to share his thoughts on retirement, he laughed.

"Why are you asking me? So far, I've retired four times and it hasn't worked yet. I'm a retirement failure and proud of it!"

Alex's first retirement came when he finished a six-year stint in the military where he learned foundational lessons of discipline and organization on which he built his following careers. One core lesson he learned: How to influence people and work with them to get things done.

After the Army, Alex attended college. He chose a teaching career for his life direction. Over the next 33 years, he modeled leadership through the education and development of young people. He moved on from being a teacher to a coach. Eventually, he rose to the position of school principal. At age 65, Alex retired for the second time. This traditional retirement most people dream about with high expectations arrived, but Alex lacked preparation for what followed.

Within three weeks, Alex had to confront the question, "What am I going to do today that will help someone?"

He felt stuck on an empty page.

"Choose something, anything!" his wife insisted.

"I think we should move. The kids have grown up and left. We no longer need this big house. Besides, it will give me something to do," he suggested.

His wife agreed. On the first day searching for a new home, they found the right size house in a perfect neighborhood. But the new home, an old house, needed lots of repairs.

Alex, now blessed with free time, embarked on what he expected would be a year and a half remodeling project. Instead, it became his third career. Word spread all over town about Alex's new project. One of his friends, bored with his retirement, requested permission to pitch in and help. This friend boasted very few carpentry skills, but he did own a pickup truck. So, Alex figured he could at least haul the trash away.

As they peeled away old wallpaper, they also uncovered a new hope about their lives and the future. Alex and his friend discovered delight and purpose in their work. As they pulled up linoleum flooring, they uncovered hardwood beneath which they sanded and refinished bringing back its original beauty. Together they experienced great fun and finished the job quickly. Eighteen months of expected work took only eight months!

When people witnessed what Alex accomplished with his own home, they started asking him to do projects for them. So, he began what became a thriving remodeling business. Walls and floors, bathrooms, kitchens, or whatever needed fixing, Alex provided. He spent the following four years doing remodeling work but then decided to retire for the third time —because a new challenge arrived.

One of Alex's former students, whom he had encouraged to attend and finish college, now shared needs with Alex concerning his expanding tech business. He thanked Alex for helping set the course for his life. Then, instead of leaving, he started a conversation about identifying people's strengths. The student described a college course in leadership that utilized the book, *Now Discover Your Strengths.*[3]

Alex's former student knew what his business needed — someone with Alex's skills and strengths. He needed someone with the ability to connect people and ideas who could encourage people to do things well.

Drinking iced tea on the front porch, Alex and his former student discussed how to grow the company. Alex's empathy and ability to sense emotions in others (an intuitive part of his nature) enabled him to understand other people's points of view, even if he didn't agree with their position. He could put himself in

---

[3] *The best way for you to quickly and deeply understand your personal strengths is through a system called Opposite Strengths. Dr. Jay Thomas and his son Dr. Tommy Thomas, both leadership psychologists and executive coaches, developed a way for you to understand your strengths, use your strengths productively, and create the best relationships you possibly can with others. Go to www.OppositeStrengths.com and read what Dr. Thomas says about "finding yourself." You can sign up for their free online strengths assessment there and get your results immediately. Then contact us here at www.dreamchapter.com – as Certified Opposite Strengths Coaches we have the expertise to coach you to apply the results in your life. And we can do that effectively either in person or online.*

their place and see the world through their eyes. The conversation led Alex to reflect on his past, especially his time in education.

The greatest delight for Alex occurred at the magic moment when a student grasped a new thought or concept, and the lightning bolt of understanding hit their brain and flashed in their eyes. He loved the joy and excitement of learning reflected back to him from his students. Alex pondered his potential to invest in more young lives. He answered the call once again to help birth creative energy in others. To him, teaching encompassed more listening than talking. Captivated by hearing stories of future hopes, Alex tapped into his gift of stirring up people to dream big dreams.

Alex found the tech world threatening, but he persevered through the challenge. His job was to be a connector — both for employees within the company and for clients. For the next 15 years, Alex remained in this position using his greatest skills every day and helping people improve their lives. Retiring again for the fourth time at the age of 88, he said, "I thought for sure this time it would stick."

But before long, Alex's phone rang with a new offer. Given his background in education and the chronic teacher shortage, he became a substitute teacher. Alex wakes every morning ready for action. Two or three days a week he gets a call to teach a class. If not needed, he goes out to his favorite places to "*connect with people.*"

Alex arises every morning intending to make the world a better place — not so much for himself, but for others. His excitement for relational growth and progress is ever-expanding. Now on his fifth career at age 90, Alex is not retired. In fact, when people ask him, Alex has a standard answer, "I don't generally cuss, but hell no! I'm not finished yet."

 Alex's primary Retirement Mindset is Wanderer.

 His secondary tendency is Seeker.

- He loves to explore possibilities (Wanderer) and search out how to help others (Seeker).
- He has the brain of a teacher.
- The attitude of an explorer.

His story is about finding joy in helping others. How would you describe your story?

Discoveries

Alex's story targets discovering purpose and meaning.

Purpose

Many people are reluctant to assess their own strengths, perhaps because of training to be humble. But take time to reflect on your life and career. Ask yourself these basic questions:

- What did you love about your career?
- What parts of your job did you most look forward to doing?
- What work accomplishments did you feel good about?
- What brought you authentic joy at work?

In retirement, the gift of time is available for investing in whatever matters most to you.

Other people tend to perceive and articulate our strengths and weaknesses better than we do. Talk to your spouse and close friends. Ask them for an honest assessment of your talents. Ask them what they think you most enjoy doing. It may be something you glossed over. Also, ask where you might improve moving forward. Alex's former student taught him a valuable lesson through their conversation on finding strengths. Your best insights may not come from yourself.

Set a Schedule

Most days Alex does the same things. He gets up and savors a cup of coffee while reading the paper. He watches the news on TV and checks to see if he is needed to teach that day. If not, Alex usually meets friends for coffee and conversation. He eats dinner around the same time every evening and goes to bed at his regularly scheduled time.

The important thing is not the specific details of Alex's schedule, but that he still stays on a schedule. People need structure and boundaries in life. Left with no externally set schedule like when working a job, most people create some kind of routine for their days. If the new schedule is not tied to something providing purpose and meaning, retirement will quickly turn to drudgery in the same way many people view work.

Keep Growing

One of the common traits of successful retirees is their search for growth opportunities. They view life as a journey moving toward new discoveries and meaningful destinations. They create excitement about something, maybe a hobby or a second job, something with a spark to capture their attention. Alex told us about one of his friends who complained about ever-changing, complicated technology while working; but after retirement, his friend improved his computer skills by taking a class on how to use technology. His negative position changed because he wanted better communication with his grandchildren.

His granddaughter did not answer phone calls or respond to voice mail. However, when he learned how to send text messages, he got instant answers. He adapted to her communication style to increase meaningful conversation. One day he provided a ride home from school for her and a few of her friends. His granddaughter exclaimed, "This is my favorite grandparent. He knows how to text!"

Lost and Found

One thing some people often miss after retirement is a title. Alex went from a lieutenant saluted to a college student, then he became a teacher and later a principal. In those early jobs, his titles provided authority and importance. In his third and fourth careers, he was just Alex. He had no authority, but something more meaningful — connections. *Connections elevate us more than titles.*

Some people find their true calling after retiring from the regular workplace. Taking time to empty yourself permits space for new discovery. Purpose changes everything. You will choose something to do. Be proactive. Let your calling find you.

You Are Meaningful

People with purpose spend no time moping around and missing their former lives. In fact, once you take the time to assess and understand yourself, including your strengths and weaknesses, you are ready to move forward. Earlier we mentioned how our culture teaches us that doing something makes us somebody. But what you are is already meaningful. Replace the notion "achievement and honor equal value." Instead tell yourself: "I am somebody. I do significant things."

You might be tempted to spend too much time staring at your trophy case of perceived life accomplishments. But don't live in the past, choose instead to focus forward rather than backward. Once you identify your strengths and interests, put them to work doing something meaningful to you now. It doesn't matter whether anyone else finds meaning in it. *It is not their retirement!*

Quest

In Alex's story, where did he find his purpose and meaning?

Where do you find purpose and meaning now?

What is the most important and powerful word people might call you?

Seed Thought

When Alex's granddaughter visited him, she pulled her mother's favorite book off the shelf. She asked her granddad to read *The Velveteen Rabbit*. When he arrived at this passage, amazement struck him at how much the children's story says about life and retirement.

"Real isn't how you are made," said the Skin Horse. "It's a thing that happens to you. When a child loves you for a long, long time, not just to play with, but REALLY loves you, then you become Real . . . . once you are Real you can't be ugly, except to people who don't understand."[4]

Perhaps the "real you" only shows up in transition.

---

[4]   Margery Williams. (1991). The Velveteen Rabbit, (New York: Delacorte Press). pp 5 – 6.

→ NOTE TO SELF

Do not let the past define you. Glance at the rearview mirror occasionally. Gaze too long and you will wreck. Let the past serve you – NOT rob you of the now!

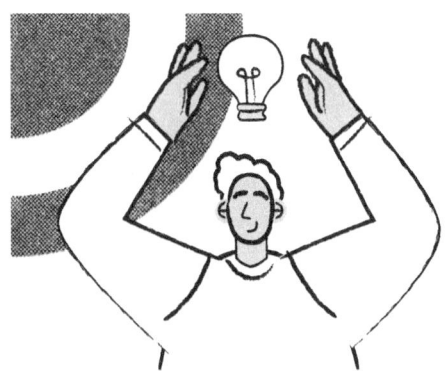

Nick the SEEKER

> *The problem with retirement is you never get a day off.*

ABE LEMONS
FORMER BASKETBALL COACH

Do you struggle to answer when people ask, "What do you do?"

Focus

Does your mental picture of retirement involve playing golf, going fishing, or enjoying a hobby all day? Sounds enticing, right? The reality is: People with nothing to live for just exist. They may pass milestones on the calendar and get older every year, but what they do can barely be called living.

Whether your dream is grand, personal, solitary, or social, if you express a desire and drive for something from your heart, you radiate life.

The opportunity to devote yourself to pursuing a dream is sometimes not found during your working career. Daily demands and responsibilities dictate how, when, where, and how long you work.

Retirement offers the chance for change, and yet, many people enter retirement without a plan leading to what is most important to them. And if nothing changes, they drift through the remaining years without experiencing the power of passion making life worthwhile. You can choose your song in advance either joining in with Peggy Lee bemoaning, "Is that all there is?" Or perhaps Kenny Rogers belting, "Let's go out in a blaze of glory." Or even better, write your own song fitting your Dream Chapter.

Nick's Journey

Nick grew up focused on the future image of himself as a major league baseball star. Adopted at birth, his parents made sacrifices to meet the needs of Nick and his adopted older sister. They encouraged Nick to play sports, but Nick eventually realized professional sports exceeded his talents. Nick then shifted his ambition to becoming a baseball coach.

Then in college, Nick shifted his aspirations to an engineering major. This choice related not to a passion for the subject, but to growing up watching the sacrifices his parents made because of financial shortfalls. His dad worked hard, but as a traveling salesman, his absence from home and limited income caused hardships.

His parents never talked about retirement. They lived from paycheck to paycheck just trying to make ends meet. In fact, they needed help from their own parents to bail them out from time to time. But they gave everything they could to their children. Nick said, "I grew up lower middle class, but my parents lived a couple of notches lower."

Nick wanted a life without economic stress, so when it came time for him to go to college, he picked a field he thought would pay well. After one semester, the differences between his interests and an engineering major became clear, so he changed his major to psychology. Like his first choice, it also failed because his decision had no root of passion, but rather grew from the hope of sufficient future income.

In August, at the beginning of his sophomore year, Nick landed a job at a local restaurant chain. By December, Nick worked his way up to the position of store manager. Nick found a perfect fit, and for the next 36 years he worked for that company, spending the last 20 of them as the president and COO. He looked forward to going to work every day and although he was not coaching sports, he did what good coaches do — build a team and help people develop the talents and skills they need to succeed.

Then Nick came to an unexpected crossroads. He wanted his own business. He hoped the owner might one day sell him the company and they began discussing the topic. The price ended up being a sticking point, and when another buyer agreed to meet the asking price, the owner changed his mind and decided not to sell the company.

Nick cashed out his share of the company and at age 55 started his own company as a franchisee of a successful restaurant brand.

He asked, "Who leverages everything at that age to start over? Someone who isn't planning to retire!"

For the next six years, Nick poured himself into growing his new business. His plan was to build until he reached a certain point, but then he received an "offer he could not refuse."

With his business sold, Nick achieved financial stability and security, but he loved working and started looking around for what to do next. He chose to become a consultant. Opportunities seemed scarce. A headhunter called with a job opening for a company that needed executive team coaching.

Soon after Nick coached his first client, another client showed up. Suddenly, Nick knew how he wanted to fill his days. He threw himself into this new career. One of his friends told him, "I haven't seen you this passionate about anything in the thirty years I've known you." Nick is now having the time of his life, fulfilling his dream. He is a retirement and leadership coach instead of a baseball coach, but he's fulfilling his passion. Nick said, "I love helping people. Sometimes I even get paid for it!"

 Nick's primary Retirement Mindset is Seeker.

- He loves to create order serving others in practical ways.
- He has the heart of a provider.
- The brain of an entrepreneur.
- The attitude of an optimist.

His story is seeking to bring quality and order to life.

What in Nick's life might bring insights into your retirement?

Discoveries

Many important lessons Nick learned did not arrive from classes or teachers, but from life. Take time. Learn from every experience.

Take Risks

Nick started over at age 55. He faced a big risk. If you are not willing to take risks, you accomplish nothing. As the old saying goes, "The turtle makes progress only when it sticks its neck out." This is not about rushing blindly without thought or planning. It requires reaching the point where after you have done due diligence, you take the first step even when the end of the trail is not visible.

It is likely some of the things you try will fail. Do not let failure stop you from trying new things. During the years Nick spent on his own business, he worked harder than ever. Taking a risk, even if it works, does not lead to coasting. Challenges may come bringing more than you think you can handle. But as hockey great Wayne Gretzky said, "You miss 100% of the shots you don't take."

Life Balance

Nick sold his business to help bring his life into better balance. He made significant investments of time into his family. His greatest pride in life is his family. Nick did not desire to work 50 to 60-hour weeks anymore. But he still wanted something to do.

Nick chose to maintain an office away from his house. This left the routines of the home intact. Retirement can have a huge impact on a spouse. His wife now could maintain her schedule without disruption. She told Nick, "I married you for better or worse — but not for lunch!" To keep things in balance requires hard work but pays great dividends.

Keep Dreaming

Nick loved his first leadership coaching job. It fueled his desire to do more. Moving forward he determined coaching would become the focus of his direction and energy. Eventually, he got another gig and then another. He searched for more opportunities to be a coach and invest in others. He had never even heard of retirement coaching which we define as "developing a non-financial retirement strategy highly meaningful for the next phase of life;" but once he discovered it, he found his natural fit.

The passion to invest in others always finds fulfillment. For some it comes in volunteering. Hospitals, libraries, schools, churches, and community groups constantly seek help. If you find one matching your talents and interests, dive in. It may be fulfilling, or it may lead you to something better when you jump the stepping-stones guiding you to forge a new direction.

Quest

What dream waiting in your heart yearns to be accomplished?

What defines your value to yourself and others?

How do "growing up" experiences still influence your life today?

Seed Thought

When Walt Disney died of cancer in 1966, construction remained in the planning stages for Disney World in Orlando, Florida. Five years later, the park opened to the public. At the opening ceremony, a reporter said to Roy Disney, "It's a shame Walt isn't here to see this." Roy Disney replied, "If Walt hadn't seen this, it wouldn't exist."

Our dreams give us a purpose and a goal for life.

Nick says, "Pursuing your dreams is what makes your retirement fulfilling."

In his poem, A *Psalm of Life*, Henry Wadsworth Longfellow wrote:

Tell me not, in mournful numbers,
    "Life is but an empty dream!"
For the soul is dead that slumbers,
    And things are not what they seem.

Life is real! Life is earnest!
    And the grave is not its goal;
"Dust thou art, to dust returnest,"
    Was not spoken of the soul.

Not enjoyment, and not sorrow,
    Is our destined end or way;
But to act, that each to-morrow
    Finds us farther than to-day.

Lives of great men all remind us
    We can make our lives sublime,
And, departing, leave behind us
    Footprints on the sands of time;

Footprints, that perhaps another,
    Sailing o'er life's solemn main,
A forlorn and shipwrecked brother,
    Seeing, shall take heart again.

Let us, then, be up and doing,
    With a heart for any fate;
Still achieving, still pursuing
    Learn to labor and to wait.

→ NOTE TO SELF

WARNING:

15 high energy years ahead
(MAYBE MORE):

Pursue your passion and transform it into

a new retirement career.

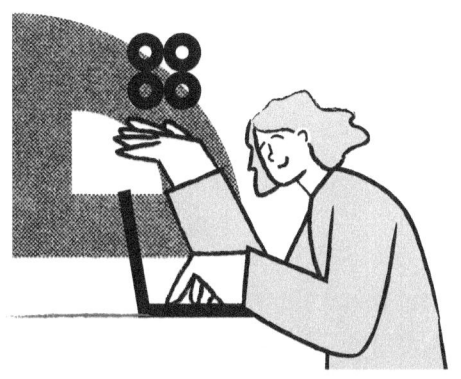

Rose the ROUTINEER

> ❝ *The real problem of leisure time is how to keep other people from using yours!*
>
> ❞
>
> ARTHUR LACEY

If the patterns of time usage you follow today become habits, what will your retirement look like?

Focus

Many people feel like they command little to no control over their lives. The workday gets scheduled around the demands of bosses, peers, and subordinates. The remaining time then fills up with obligations to family, community, hobbies, church, neighborhood groups, and other interests. Most people feel like they have little control of their time. With the transition to retirement, many of those time demands go away leaving some people poorly equipped about how to fill their time.

The outcome of your retirement, whether it lives up to your dreams and expectations or not, will be determined by how you use your time.

We often speak of "spending" time, the perfect analogy, since time is a precious resource and once gone, it can never be recovered. That is why the 51% Principle is so important. As we go through Rose's story, you'll see what this means and how it matters in successful retirement.

Rose's Journey

I met with Rose a few months before her planned retirement. In thirty-two years with her company, she rose to the top, becoming one of the first African American CEOs in her industry. One of the great things about coaching is the opportunity to learn more than you teach. Such proved to be true in my conversations with Rose.

As I often do, I asked, "What do we need to talk about today in your preparation for retirement?"

Rose replied, "We need to talk about what a typical week will look like a year from now. I'm only six months away from retirement, and I'm thinking a lot about how life will go. What are the surprises and landmines I need to avoid? What could potentially keep me from obtaining the retirement I want?"

We talked for a few moments about her current schedule. As the CEO of the company, Rose faced many demands and expectations.

The company set a time for the workday to start, and as she pointed out, the board expected the CEO to lead by example and arrive at work on time. The schedule for the daily lunch break was set by corporate policy. And while an official quitting time existed, eight hours of work never got everything done. She worked many weekends after working 10-to-12-hour days during the week.

Then Rose said, "I realize looking back at it now, regarding my schedule, the company basically ran my life for 32 years. That stops on the first morning after my retirement."

I asked her to close her eyes and picture a day in retirement with her schedule under her control. "How would that look?" I asked. "More importantly, how would it feel?"

Her first response was, "I'm not setting the alarm. I'll get up when I wake up!"

The length of her commute to work dictated the time for her to get up for many years. She talked about the joy of sitting on the back porch enjoying a cup of coffee with no stressful demands. One high priority for her was *to spend quality time with her young grandchildren.* For years she had longed to give them more personalized attention, but her work schedule constrained her. Rose's husband also planned several things he hoped they could do together. She had put off several good organizations asking her for help by saying, "When I retire. And now they are reminding me of it!"

As we talked about how things would be different in retirement and how she would allocate her time, I introduced her to the 51% Principle. I first came across this concept in 1995 through the book of the same name by Dr. William Lantz and Connie Lantz.[5] The central concept is built around the analogy of corporate ownership. Picture your life being represented by 100 shares of stock. You own 51% of the shares. That means you own the power to make choices.

None of us owns complete control. The other 49% of your life is owned by others — spouse, children, parents, bosses, employees, neighbors, and many others with input on how to invest your time, energy, and resources. Many people can place legitimate demands on your time and attention. But in the final

---

[5]   William C. Lantz and Connie S. Lantz. (1995). *The Fifty-One Percent Principle: Taking Control over Your Life.* Tulsa, OK: Honor Books.

analysis, you are the majority "stockholder". The big decisions fall on you. The 51% Principle is about accountability reminding you who gets to choose. Decisions *you* make (or fail to make) determine how your retirement goes.

You are the majority shareholder of your own retirement. You would never think of making serious financial investments without thought and careful attention. Yet many people treat an even more valuable resource than money, *their time*, in a very casual fashion. They do not stop to deeply consider what they want to accomplish. As a result, their time and energy are spent on things unable to bring happiness, create value, or leave something important behind.

Rose chose a simple goal. Here are the two questions that helped her identify and specify her goal:

> When you start wrapping up life on this earth, what do you want people to remember about you?
>
> What did your family members do for you in your formative years that you want to pass on?

She didn't hesitate for a second. "I received the gift of specialness."

Rose told me about an aunt who, having no children of her own, took Rose into her heart.

"She gave me the gift of love for reading and learning. She raised lavender in her flower beds from which she would make perfume. I can still remember sitting in her lap while she read to me as I breathed in her words and her sweet lavender aroma. She believed in me and treated me like I was very special. That made all the difference in my life."

Rose wants to provide the same feeling to her grandchildren.

"They are special. I tell their mothers intellectual capital skips a generation! We laugh about it, but they are special, and the world won't tell them that. They need to experience the rich internal feeling for themselves so they can believe it."

She leaned back laughing and said, "I can't wait to retire from this job and start scheduling those moments of specialness in my life."

I experienced an "ah-ha" moment when Rose said, "In my family, I don't have any role models for making the transition into retirement."

She became the first in her family to ever retire. No one before her accumulated the resources to stop working. I helped her blaze a trail into uncharted territory. It felt like walking on sacred ground. We both realized she would be leaving behind an example for others to follow.

Knowing she blazed a trail for future generations caused Rose to focus even more intensely on the priorities of designing her new plans. For her, this was serious business. So, I asked Rose two more questions:

> What do you want to target in the first four to five years of retirement?

> How can you allocate your time and resources to make sure you hit the target?

Working out answers to these questions, I said, "Rose, you've grasped the 51% Principle. You are owning your future. Now it is up to you."

A wasted life is nothing more than a lot of wasted days piled together.

As you think about replacing your work schedule with a retirement schedule, consider what you really want to accomplish, what commitments you must make to accomplish those things, and how you retain control of your life. Choose not to be a victim. You have the power to change things. Keep your 51% "ownership shares". Retain your choices and take responsibility for *your* retirement.

 Rose's primary Retirement Mindset is Routineer.

 Her secondary tendency is Planner.

- She loves to establish order out of chaos.
- She has the brain of an accountant.
- She has a heart for creating community.
- The attitude of a caring provider.

Her story is discovering how to manage life priorities and time.

How do you plan to spend your "best time" in retirement?

Discoveries

A New Kind of Accountability

During our employment career, we are held accountable in a variety of ways. Most of us start out punching a time clock. Over time we move up in the company but still report to managers, boards, and shareholders who expect results and accountability. Successful people hold themselves accountable to a high degree without regard to outside factors. In the working world, defined standards of accountability are clear. But what about retirement? Who holds you accountable?

Accountability starts by formulating specific goals. Without a standard of measurement, it is difficult to judge progress. Vastly different targets now challenge you than in the workplace. For example, I told Rose one thing she needed to be accountable for was scheduling time for relaxing. If you worked for years in the "fast lane", slowing down and recharging the batteries can be a challenge, but it is vital. Take note, it is not just relaxing — it is intentional relaxation. It is not loafing through life, but rather taking time to rest so you can do more of what you want.

It's Not Too Late

Rose felt guilt over not spending more time with her grandchildren. The demands of being CEO of a large company made it impossible for her to make the impact on their young lives like she desired. You may have similar feelings about making an impact. But good news, you can start making a change today. Determine what time in your schedule you need for accomplishing the things of highest value to you.

At retirement, Rose's three grandchildren were ages 4 to 7. She was fortunate. That is prime time for creating special bonding moments and making lifetime memories. But if you missed the early years, start today. Go forward from the present with intentional resolve to accomplish your set goals.

When the Pressure's Off

Rose found one part of the transition difficult. She said, "I've tried to think how it will feel without the stress and pressure of answering to others. I felt constantly compelled to do my best for the board, the stockholders, and our employees who were counting on me."

It concerned her how she would react when all the outside pressure turned off. By the way, she did just fine!

This is where the 51% Principle enters. When you take ownership, you don't need someone on the outside to provide the pressure to keep going. You take accountability for yourself, and you provide the necessary impetus. Sure, if you need extra rest, go back to bed. But if not, get up and get on with the good things in front of you. You do not need someone standing over you or creating standards for you to enjoy a good retirement.

How You Start Matters a LOT

One thing tripping up some people is how they handle the first days and weeks of retirement. The patterns you start and set during this transition become habits impacting the next twenty or thirty-plus years. In retirement, success becomes easier if you begin right. You absolutely can change tracks if you start off wrong, but it is more difficult. Life is path dependent and once an original path is created, it is not easy to abandon and create a fresh start.

Rose's success in retirement is a perfect example of the importance of planning your schedule and priorities ahead of time. It did not take months or years to start down the path. She already knew where she wanted to arrive and how she planned to get there. She did not waste her time. Do not overlook the importance of good habits in retirement.

The Paradox of Choice

Take time to review your work career. For the first ten years of work, you probably had little say in how you spent your time. Tasks were assigned and given deadlines. Often the method of carrying out those tasks was dictated by others. Over time, most people find more freedom to choose where and how to spend their time. While it might seem more choices make things easier, the fact is — it usually makes things more complicated.

As Rose moved up in the company, she did not think about the stress of excess choices and insufficient time. But after a few years at the top, she decided to retire, in part because of the impact of stress on her health. Retirement offers a great variety of choices, usually more choices for you to make than in your working career. It is important to have a clear destination in mind, not just to help you arrive, but also to reduce the stress of choosing from so many options. Live in the moment. Reach for reasons to celebrate. Refuse to be confined by what others think of you. And treat each day as a gift to be unwrapped.

Quest

Did anyone in your family model a plan of intentional retirement for you?

If not, how can you leave a good retirement road map to those who come after you?

Have you given away ownership of your life to others rather than taking control?

Seed Thought

Perhaps your life to this point has not been lived by the 51% Principle. Maybe you allowed other people control over your choices. Reverse that! Take responsibility and accountability for yourself. Take back control. One of the most renowned and famous businessmen in history, Steve Jobs, dropped out of college to co-found Apple Computers. The company made him famous and wealthy, but at 30 years of age the board of directors forced him out of leadership.

Jobs admittedly floundered in 1985 without his job. He told the graduates of Stanford University, "I didn't know what to do for a few months. I felt that I had let the previous generation of entrepreneurs down, that I had dropped the baton as it was being passed to me. I even thought about running away from (Silicon) Valley. But something slowly began to dawn on me. I still loved what I did. The turn of events at Apple had not changed that one bit. And so, I decided to start over."

Twelve years later in 1997, it was Apple's turn for floundering, and Steve Jobs was called back as CEO to turn things around. Over the next few years, the iPod, iPhone, and iPad revolutionized the computing and communications world. Jobs said, "I didn't see it then, but it turned out that getting fired from Apple was the best thing that could have ever happened to me. I'm pretty sure none of this would have happened if I hadn't been fired from Apple. It was awful tasting medicine, but I guess the patient needed it. Sometimes life hits you in the head with a brick. Don't lose faith. I'm convinced the only thing that kept me going was that I loved what I did. You've got to find what you love."

And once you find what you love, take responsibility for making it happen.

Your retirement WILL be a success if you take responsibility and love what you do.

→ **NOTE TO SELF**

Slow down. Roll down the windows. Don't miss the beauty and the fragrance of the world around you. Share the grand places with the grandchildren.

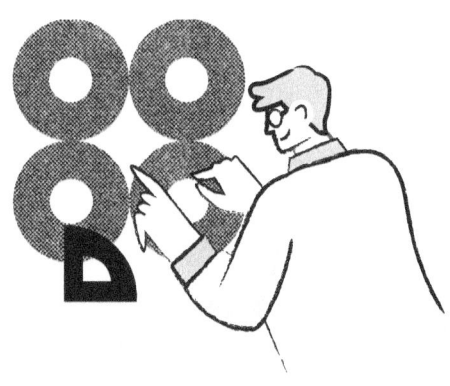

Ethan the PLANNER

"After all these years,
why don't you retire
and go fishing?"
*"I would but the fish
don't applaud."*

BOB HOPE

What if the most threatening problem to retirement enjoyment is something you control?

Focus

In 2020, the life expectancy of a 65-year-old male was 17.4 years and for a 65-year-old female it was 20.1 years. With an additional 20 years at age 65, we need to focus on maintaining our health and vitality. Those able to remain active and well enjoy a far higher quality of life than those who become inactive. While certain genetic and environmental factors impact health, the fact remains: much of our health, both now and in the future, falls under our control.[6]

The well-being you enjoy or endure in retirement rests, in part, with your active choice to protect and promote health starting now.

---

[6] Life expectancy data is from "Provisional Life Expectancy Estimates for 2020", *Vital Statistics Rapid Release, Report No. 015, July 2021.* Accessed at cdc.gov/nchs/data/vsrr/vsrr015-508.pdf on 11/27/21.

Ethan's Journey

Ethan grew up in a small community. Driving fifty miles or more every time he needed to see a doctor affected his childhood. Never did this impact him more than when he found himself chasing his friends along a path in the woods. Ethan held the unfortunate spot in the line of laughing children who had stirred up the wrath of a large rattlesnake. The snake struck. His personal pain and the fear exhibited on the faces of his parents during the long trip to the nearest emergency medical facility with antivenin helped influence him at a young age to become a doctor in a rural community. After many years of education, Ethan set up his practice in a small town, becoming "the" doctor everyone around needed, and he enjoyed a successful career.

After he retired, he reached out to me for retirement coaching. We met for lunch, and I asked him some questions about his life before and after retirement. We did a Retirement Assessment Inventory to make sure we knew where he currently stood and where he wanted to be in the future. As we continued, it became clear — the primary goal for Ethan was self-care.

As a doctor, Ethan had encyclopedic knowledge about how the mind and body work. But like many medical professionals, he did not put that knowledge to work in his own life.

The things we do, not the things we know, determine our outcome.

Ethan kept up to date on all the latest studies and findings, but he could not muster the discipline to do the right things.

Ethan lived under a job loaded with stress. However, the reality of the modern world is that most jobs deliver high stress levels. Expectations and demands on our time easily take control of our lives. Often our response to stress is unhealthy. People may eat too much or eat the wrong things, get less sleep, or perhaps overuse alcohol or medication in attempts to cope with stress.

For Ethan, losing weight and strengthening his body rose to first place on his list for self-improvement. Looking at him, I did not think he was overweight. But as we talked, he introduced me to a new term: "skinny fat". His fat to muscle ratio was out of balance. So, Ethan's plan contained not a specific diet but changing lifelong habits to strengthen his body. Success would not be measured on the scale of weight loss, but of strength gained.

The average American male gains one pound per year starting at the age of 25. The slow gain takes a long time to notice, but when people reach their 40s and 50s, the expansion shows. Ethan planned to slowly lose the weight he gained over the years at one pound per month. He designed a pattern of nutrition and exercise to follow for the rest of his life.

Rather than cutting food intake, he changed his food consumption. He ate fewer sugary foods, replacing them with natural foods. He also cut down on fatty meat and added more healthy protein to his meals. Every person is different and needs a personalized approach. The important thing is having a plan that works for you.

Ethan quoted Yogi Berra, **"If you don't know where you're going, you will wind up somewhere else."**

Start early. It is easier to control weight and build strength at fifty than at sixty, and easier at forty than at fifty. If you think ahead and take care of your health including body, mind, and spirit, you will experience a better retirement. It will come as no surprise, given his many years in the medical profession, but Ethan emphasized the importance of going to the doctor for the best source of information about your specific nutrition and exercise plan.

 Ethan's primary Retirement Mindset is Planner.

 His secondary tendency is Routineer.

- He loves to care for the health issues of others.
- He has the heart of a caregiver.
- The brain of a knowledgeable researcher.
- The attitude of a learner.

His story is focusing on others to the point of not taking care of himself.

Why is health care important to you?

Discoveries

Sleep Heals

As the only doctor in a small farming community, emergency calls during the night frequently interrupted Ethan's slumber. This created unhealthy sleep patterns. This problem began in medical school and carried on in odd working hours during residency. Ethan confessed, "I did not understand what the human body needs in regard to sleep and even what I did know I did not put into practice." Research shows sleep to be an extremely important factor to health, memory, and enjoyment of life. Such bedrock truth holds both before and after retirement!

Things in life easily get out of control. Ethan could not choose when the phone rang at night during his working career. But he changed the things he could like taking the television set out of the bedroom. He lowered the temperature in the house at night to promote deeper sleep. Rapid eye movement (REM) sleep proves critical to both physical and mental health. Without it, sickness, irritability, and anxiety increase. In the words of the six-fingered man, Count Rugen, to Prince Humperdinck in *The Princess Bride*, "Get some rest. If you haven't got your health, you haven't got anything."

Schedule Your Exercise

Ethan intended to exercise, but due to the daily pressures of his medical practice, he struggled and failed. Preparing for a health-focused retirement, he decided to schedule walks first thing in the morning. He could control his schedule better earlier in the day since emergency calls occur less frequently in the early hours. He began gently, just walking around the block. Then he lengthened his walks. He increased his walks to thirty minutes a day, gradually increasing the speed of his pace. Soon he noticed improvement in his mental alertness and his energy level throughout the day.

He also scheduled training with a yoga instructor. Learning basic stretches improved his flexibility. Gerontology research indicates pneumonia as a leading cause of death among retirees, behind heart disease and cancer. Many cases of pneumonia follow a fall and a broken bone leading to inactivity and confinement. Regularly working to improve flexibility helps prevent falls and helps with posture.

Drink More Water

The human body is 60% water. Water is vital to the healthy functioning of cells. Few people drink water in the amount the human body needs.

Ethan said, "I found I must be intentional about water intake. The older I get the easier it becomes to not think about it." Increasing water consumption requires building new habits and discipline.

While the amount of water needed varies by person, health studies promote the benefits of 64 ounces per day — drinking an 8-ounce glass of water 8 times. Dehydration negatively impacts physical energy, stamina, and mental functions. Research indicates increased water consumption also promotes weight loss.

Don't Go Solo

Do not overlook the need for community and interaction with others in retirement. Our health is affected by being around other healthy people. They challenge you to "up your game" and encourage you to develop good health habits.

Ethan said, "I choose to spend most of my time with friends who are proactive about life instead of those who are stuck in anger or believe their best days are over."

In retirement, it is not unusual for a spouse to be diagnosed with a debilitating illness. Unfortunately, research reveals many caretakers die before the one needing special care. If you find yourself in a caretaker role, get help. Balance your time by spending as much time as possible with energetic grandchildren and healthy friends. Your love for life will lighten your spouse's spirits.

Obviously, aging requires significant adjustments. No matter how healthy or focused we are, the body can no longer do all it once did. But spending time with others who are focused on health helps you maintain your commitment and provides encouragement and interaction. Someone wisely pointed out, "The Lone Ranger wasn't!" The masked man's "faithful companion", Tonto, stayed by his side.

Spiritual Health Matters

Refrain from thinking of spiritual health only in a religious sense. While religion may be part of it, the focus of spirituality is more about your inward being. Worry and stress tend to overwhelm and literally take your thoughts captive. Ethan found freedom by forming a nightly habit of reviewing his day and focusing his attention on something (or someone) causing the uplift of a grateful spirit within him. In addition to reducing his stress level, Ethan said, "Gratitude impacted my attitude. I began expecting good things to happen."

We desire meaning and purpose in life. Maintaining spiritual and physical health makes it easier to find meaning and purpose in our retirement years. Enjoy your unique gift of life. Nothing is guaranteed. As a summation of a healthy spiritual attitude, the Serenity Prayer is as good as it gets:

"Lord, give me the serenity to accept the things I cannot change, the courage to change the things I can, and the wisdom to know the difference."

Synergy

Ethan said, "The body works as a whole unit, and synergistic power comes into play as you put these pieces of self-care together. Movement is life. Action causes reaction. Being outside increases the natural intake of vitamin D. Walking or running increases thirst. Exercise releases natural endorphins which make you think and feel better. These internal chemicals act as painkillers improving your sleep and reducing stress. As a matter of fact, each health improvement you choose to bring into play reinforces and builds on the others."

Choices

"Which form of exercise is best? Swimming? Biking? Running? Brisk walking? Tennis? Dancing?" I asked.

Ethan replied, "Whichever one you enjoy the most!"

Quest

If your health continues its current trajectory, where do you expect to be in five years?

Do you have a regularly scheduled and consistent exercise program?

What one change might you make in your life today to improve your physical, mental and spiritual health?

Seed Thought

Mickey Mantle, one of the best baseball players of all time, made the All-Star Team 16 times, played in 12 World Series with the Yankees, winning 7 of them, and still holds many offensive records. Mantle three times won the MVP of the American League. He famously dueled with teammate Roger Maris in the home run hitting season of 1961, falling just short of Babe Ruth's season record (and finishing behind

Maris). Despite his incredible athletic gifts, Mantle died at just 63 years of age.

In 1994, 25 years after his baseball career ended, and after decades of heavy drinking, he checked into the Betty Ford Clinic and embraced sobriety. But the damage to his body could not be reversed. Despite receiving a liver transplant in June 1995, Mantle died in August. He declared a truth we all need the wisdom and discipline to apply: "If I'd known I was going to live this long, I'd have taken a lot better care of myself."

Consequently, take care of *your* health. Fully enjoy retirement incorporating a health-focused balance with family, friends, and hobbies. Don't wait until it's too late to start improving. **Choose today to activate plans to powerfully impact years yet to come.** Choose to live healthy!

NOTE TO SELF

He who manages a fleet of trucks and fails due to laziness or a busy schedule to care for his own vehicle is not wise. Yes, Dr. Do Little Exercise, practice what you preach starting today!

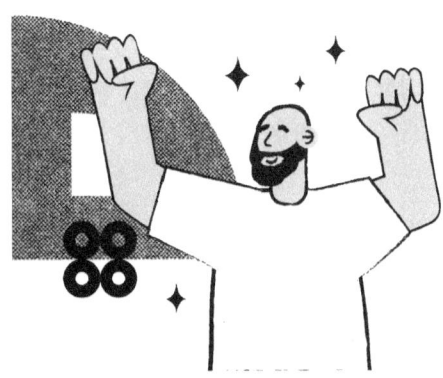

Ted the **ROUTINEER**

" *Unhappy is he who depends on success to be happy. In this case, there will not be life after success.* **"**

ALEX DIAS RIBERO
FORMER FORMULA 1 DRIVER

What one thing can you completely control in both preparing for and living out your retirement years?

Focus

Many things in life fall within your influence such as improving your health by taking care of your body or improving your finances by taking care of your money. In addition, you might improve your location by deciding where to live. And the possibility exists for you to improve the value of your time by what you put on or take off your calendar. People think they control these areas of life, but upon closer inspection, none of us can totally control any of them. Other people and things beyond our control play a huge role in outcomes.

One thing that you own complete and total control over is ATTITUDE. Attitude is a mindset experience. You can choose how you will respond before something happens. Decide in advance to look for the best response no matter what transpires. Is the glass half full or half empty? We all know the same amount of liquid is in it, yet we often forget the choice of perspective is up to us. We alone control which approach we take.

Ted's Journey

Ted's entire career was in the banking business. He reached the position of CEO in his early fifties and aimed to retire at age 67. At his retirement party, one of his friends gave him the gift of retirement coaching, bringing me into the picture.

We sat down together for our first session one week after his official retirement day. He had no expectation about the retirement coaching process, and since I had never met him before, neither of us knew what to expect. The first session was delightful. I enjoyed getting to know him. He shared his history and his greatest memories about work, family, and community involvement. We set up a time for our second appointment.

When we met the second time, I was shocked. I had never seen a bigger change in a person in such a short time frame. Ted's facial expressions and body language completely altered, and not in a good way.

"We planned to talk today about new routines and schedules. Is that what we need to talk about?" I asked him.

With a grim look on his face, Ted responded, "Not really." His elegant and expressive communication style in our first meeting was gone. Ted squirmed awkwardly in his chair.

"I don't know exactly how to put this into words," he said.

"How are you feeling?" I asked.

"Terrible," he replied. "I think something is wrong with me physically, and I'm going to make an appointment with my doctor. I saw him six months ago and everything was fine."

"Describe your feelings and how they are showing up," I said.

"No energy. I'm sleeping a lot. I've lost my appetite. I find myself irritated by small things," Ted responded. "My wife announced our grandkids were coming over to spend the night with us and I got angry. That's not me at all. I love my grandkids. I know something is wrong with me. I'm constantly tired."

I asked him, "How would you describe your attitude?"

"Low at times. Angry at times. Highly frustrated at times. Fearful at times. It seems like I've lost control of my feelings," he admitted.

"Have you ever had this kind of mindset before?" I asked.

"Not really. I've had all these emotions, but only briefly. Now it seems like I'm living permanently in this despondent attitude of life. Do you think something is wrong with me?" he asked.

I avoided the answer and said, "Let's keep talking. If you were coaching me and I told you what you just said, what would you tell me to do?"

He laughed, "I'd tell you to go see the doctor and find out what was going on. Obviously, I need to make that doctor's appointment. As soon as I find out the results from my physical, we'll have our next session."

Three weeks later we scheduled a time to meet. Session three started with his health report, which showed no significant physical problems causing his symptoms.

"So how would you describe your attitude now?" I asked.

"I'm still having a tough time, but it's not as bad as it was. I still don't like life right now," he said.

"Could I walk you through an exercise I think will help?" I asked.

"Of course," he replied.

I asked him to write down the following.

Life Event + Response / Reaction = Outcome

"Which of the three elements in this equation can you control?" I asked.

He thought for a little bit and then said, "Only the middle part. I choose whether to respond or react to what happens."

"Explain the difference between response and reaction," I requested.

"Reaction tends to complain, blame, and criticize. That's ugly. I have blamed others for what I'm feeling," he confessed. "Response tries to find a solution."

"What bothers you the most since retiring?" I asked.

"Well, not one single person from the bank has called me since I retired. They haven't asked for my opinion about anything related to the business. Do they think I got stupid when I retired?"

"When did you become CEO?" I asked.

"I remember it well, I was 52," he answered.

"Who did you replace?" I asked.

He named the man holding the post before him.

"Did you ever call him in the first couple months and ask for his advice?" I asked.

"No, I didn't want to bother him," he *paused*. A new perspective suddenly came to Ted. "Oh," he moaned.

I continued, "You told yourself the story 'I am no longer valued.' You missed the more probable story. They don't want to bother you."

"I like your story much better than mine," he said.

"Retirement is a major life event. Things change. The future is determined by whether we respond or react. You can tell yourself a negative story. You can tell yourself a positive story.

Control is yours. One is a reaction, and the other is a response. Were you a problem solver during your career or a complainer?" I asked.

"I loved solving problems," he answered.

"When negative emotions well up in you, stop and ask yourself, are you responding or reacting? Let's talk again in two weeks. Put this card where you can see it every morning," I instructed.

I handed him the card. "Put one word over the plus sign. PAUSE."

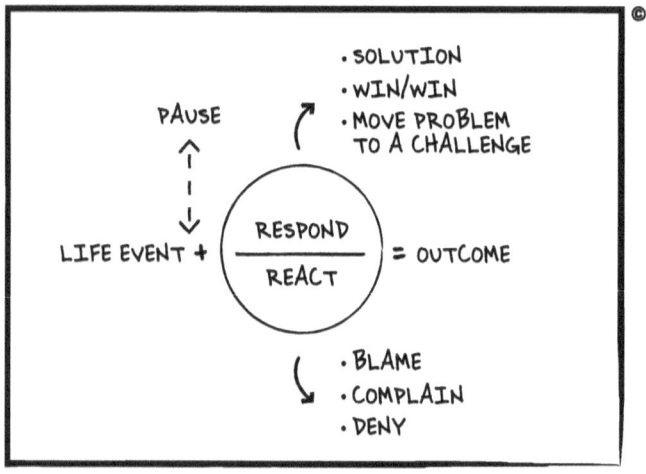

Attitude is a choice. Ted's journey began by finding adjustments to his attitude.

I planned to start Session Four with the same question, "How are you feeling?"

Ted entered the room with a big smile on his face. The first thing he said was, "I can't wait to tell you about the change I've experienced."

"I can't wait to hear it," I replied.

"I got it."

"What?"

"A week after our last session I went to a Rotary meeting. The speaker talked about how attitude determines altitude. All of us face downers. It's not the downers but how we choose to respond or react that makes the difference. Do you know how pearls are made? An irritated oyster. They get a grain of sand inside their shell, and to stop it from causing pain they coat it with a smoothing substance they created from within them that makes a pearl. They adjust to the irritation and a positive response creates value. I experienced my breakthrough when I realized what I'm getting irritated about needs a response, not a reaction. I need to find the good side and tell myself a new story," said Ted.

That was three years ago. Ted is now investing in his life, his family, and his community. He is a joy to be around. His present positive attitude viewing his retirement years as a gift has changed other people as well. Ted makes a positive impact because of his attitude.

 Ted's primary Retirement Mindset is Routineer.

 His secondary tendency is Planner.

- He loves to enjoy the moment.
- He has the brain of a mathematician.
- He has the heart of an entertainer.
- The attitude of a challenger.

His story is one of adjusting to retirement.

What is your toughest adjustment in retirement?

Discoveries

Pause that Refreshes

Choice usually comes at the beginning. Avoid letting false mental constructs send your emotions out of orbit. *Pause* works as your escape hatch. Whether you face a bad medical diagnosis, financial reversals, or relationship breaks, you still own control. Seek a solution allowing you to produce pearls of great value.

Patience Drives Attitude

Patience is a key driver of attitude. Patience is not simply the ability to wait but the ability to retain a positive outlook while waiting for the best.

Join Other Positive People

Spending time with other positive people charges your positive attitude battery. Your associates catch the attitude you project, and you tend also to reflect or absorb their attitude. Intentionally and carefully choose the people with whom you hang out. Attitude is caught more often than it is taught.

Expect the Best

For one entire week try to go without complaining about anything or blaming anyone for anything. Good luck! Start a habit of replacing negative thinking with positive thinking. Pause, respond, and seek the good in any event.

Live in the Present Moment

Refuse to focus on what went wrong in the past. Likewise, refuse to worry about what might go wrong in the future. You cannot control the past. It is over. Let it go. You cannot totally control the future so do not let brooding about the future rob you of the good in the present.

Quest

In retirement, what bothers you the most?

Can you pause and choose another perspective?

How might you take irritations and create pearls?

Seed Thought

Victor Frankl, Austrian neurologist, psychiatrist, philosopher, author, and holocaust survivor spoke richly about the sphere of reality encompassing choices we have for creating a better response to our present situations.[7]

"Between stimulus and response there is a space. In that space is our power to choose our response. In our responses lies our growth and our freedom."

Victor Frankl lived for over four years in Nazi concentration camps. In a way, he turns us inside out with realities too difficult for us to understand, except that all people get a taste of suffering during their lives. Whether it is a taste, or a meal, or years of suffering, Frankl's message to us is insightful. *Even when you have no ability to change your circumstances, the challenge is to change yourself.*

---

[7]   Victor Frankl authored many insightful books dealing with the meaning of life. Among his books are *Yes to Life: In Spite of Everything and Man's Search for Meaning*. Reading any of his books will be time well spent.

NOTE TO SELF

Let yourself be surprised by joy at the unexpected detours.

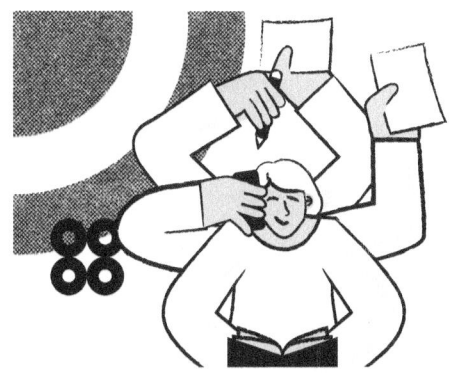

Tracy the SEEKER

"

*Often when
you think you are at the
end of something, you are
at the beginning of
something else.*

"

FRED ROGERS

Right now, what can you start, stop, or continue doing to bring the greatest value to life?

Focus

Meaning and purpose in life differ from person to person. Take time to analyze your life to determine what is most important to you. But regardless of your specific discoveries concerning success and meaning, none of them are restricted to a job or a paycheck. They relate more to your personal values and how you choose to spend your time.

You will not find deep meaning in your life if you fail to look for it. If you aim at nothing, you're sure to hit it.

Transitioning into retirement with a financial plan, but without a life meaning plan is like flying a jumbo jet with no destination. A life meaning plan enables your retirement jet to smoothly touch down on the right runway at the right airport! Make sure your time, talents, energy, and resources are packed carefully into the things that really matter to you. Defining your meaning and purpose is crucial to transitioning into a happy and productive retirement.

Tracy's Journey

In her corporate career, Tracy steadily rose through the ranks of a large professional firm. She moved from one key leadership role to the next as her skills and passion allowed her to succeed with larger and broader areas of responsibility. Over the course of working with Tracy during her career, we identified five key measures of success helping her focus on what really mattered to her. Every person's list differs depending on the boundaries of their talents, goals, and experiences. Tracy's list:

1. *The Principle of Influence*: Your influence impacts others to the degree you place their interests first. Give attention.
2. *The Principle of Others*: Every person you meet is worthy of your best. Give respect.

3. *The Principle of Vision*: Always help others see the promise of a better tomorrow. Give hope.
4. *The Principle of Positivity*: When life presents roadblocks, find a way to keep moving forward. Give courage.
5. *The Principle of Mission*: Live a life of integrity with emphasis on relationships. Give yourself.

Tracy retired at age 58. I knew her well and was chosen to speak at her retirement party. By anyone's measure, she achieved success. But most importantly, Tracy succeeded in what mattered most to her. With her permission, I shared these principles with the large gathering. I saw smiles of recognition throughout the room as people heard familiar phrases and expressions. In fact, she had them printed on cards and shared them with young executives she mentored. Even years after her retirement, you could still find the cards with *Tracy's Success Index* all around the building.

In the two years of planning and preparing for her retirement, Tracy realized: None of her five key principles depend on being employed or drawing a paycheck. They transitioned perfectly to retirement. Setting clear goals and measures of success is not just for corporate executives. It matters for parents, teachers, mechanics, ranchers, coaches, janitors, pastors, and doctors. It matters to everyone.

If you have no specific goals in mind, you will drift into the end of your life with needless regrets. Take time to find your "sweet spot" so you know what matters most to you, then establish a plan to succeed in those areas. During our two years working together, we did not focus primarily on financial planning. Instead, we focused on planning for life — how Tracy might live so her unique success index would continue to guide her days.

As part of that process, we used a set of three elements contributing to an identification of focus: passion/purpose, strengths/constraints, and values/priorities.

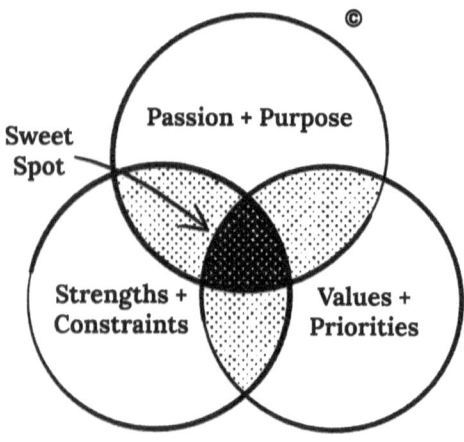

Most people find this process uncomfortable, especially the part about strengths and constraints. Tracy found it very awkward. She found it easier to list what she did not do well (the Constraints) than to list what she did well (the Strengths). But we took the time to work through the process. When you find the places where those elements overlap, you have identified areas to focus on which, in turn, produce the greatest results and impact, in your life and in the lives of others.

Tracy said, "This process helped me more than I expected. I learned my mission does not change in retirement. What drives me and brings me delight is trying to help others — particularly helping them to live productive lives. My life purpose energizes me with a powerful passion to roll out of bed every morning and do it all over again."

Often, people entering retirement fail to grasp the significant increase in choices and control over the use of their time. In a full-time job, much of your time is directed and controlled by other people, those you report to and those who report to you. You may offer input into goals and tasks, but often those are formulated by others; sometimes without your participation at all. Subsequently, you may not be the one to define and delineate the priorities and measures of success.

In retirement, the tide turns. You now determine goals, tasks, direction, and purpose. And success requires intentionality about the content of your days.

One year after retirement, Tracy said, "The prep work we did really paid off. What a wonderful year! I am here for a purpose. My passion finds fulfillment now more than ever. I get to invest in other people's lives, especially young people. I appreciate every minute I have for doing what I love most."

Identification of your strengths, values, and priorities helps you focus your efforts. But seeing the vision is only the beginning — you also must develop a strategy able to take you where you want to go. For example, one goal for Tracy was building relationships. Relationships mattered far more to her than having a job title.

In fact, Tracy said, "I love it when someone introduces me as 'my friend' Tracy. That's far better than being called 'my boss' Tracy."

Having identified the value of relationships, Tracy focuses on her sweet spot — investing in other people. When she wakes up in the morning, no one instructs her what to do. The choices for the use of her time and energy belong to her.

Looking back on her working career, Tracy carries few regrets. But she shared one.

"If I could go back in time, I would invest more time in fewer people rather than the investment of a little time with a lot of people. Surface relationships produce such small impact," she said.

If your life is consumed by maneuvering from one task to the next — whether in your work career or in retirement — you will likely miss opportunities to do what matters most to you.

Another thing Tracy discovered in her adjustment to retirement included the kindness of saying "No." Unless you can say no to the options outside of your personal sweet spot, you lose the ability to say "Yes" to the ones you want. Many good and worthy causes exist, but there is only one you. Preparing for retirement attuned Tracy's mind and spirit, not just in making the adjustments from working life, but in focusing on what matters most to her now. Focusing narrows things down. Only the narrow way hits the center of the target.

"I found a special peace and joy in my retirement. It motivates me to stay attentive not only to others but to how I take care of myself physically, mentally, and emotionally so that I can keep on living this meaningful life I love of serving others!" said Tracy.

Tracy's primary Retirement Mindset is Seeker.

 Her secondary tendency is Planner.

- She loves to make a difference in impacting others' thinking.
- She has the brain of an evaluator.
- She has the heart of a champion.
- The attitude of a "difference maker."

Her story is one of where and how to invest her interest, commitment, and time.

What is the success "sweet spot" for you in retirement?

Discoveries

Overcome Constraints Through Reverse Mentoring

We gravitate to thinking of mentoring as something flowing from an experienced older person to the younger, but it also works wonderfully in the other direction. For example, the assessment we did of strengths and constraints with Tracy revealed her to be weak in keeping up with new technology and communication. She could have been inclined to stick with the comfortable and ignore continual advances.

Instead, she found a young person fluent in "tech-speak" to teach her about the power of phones, tablets, and computers. New skills matter because Tracy values relationships. She needs the ability to communicate effectively with people in whom she hopes to invest her time. You may find you need a savvy youngster to help maximize your efficiency in whatever you choose to do in retirement.

Be Open to Things You Have Not Considered

We focused until now in this story on the importance of spending your time and energy primarily on things you identify as being in your personal sweet spot. But stay alert for surprise exceptions to the rule. You may stumble upon your sweet spot in places never imagined. For Tracy, that meant saying "Yes" to a friend who asked her to spend half a day at a local blood drive.

"The only reason I agreed to this queasy adventure was because of my friendship with Sarah. The idea of blood drives attracted no interest or passion for me at all," said Tracy.

But Tracy found delight in meeting the people and helping keep everything organized.

"Okay, Sarah," she said. "This wasn't as painful as I expected. I'll be back again next week to help."

Soon it developed into a regular part of Tracy's schedule, and now every week she is in town she spends at least half a day helping with the blood drive. Her passions, strengths, and values overlapped for a perfect fit. But had she not been willing to try something new — she would have completely missed it.

Take Responsibility for Time Management Transitions

Retirement, especially from a job with high expectations and demands, permits you a respite from the stress of producing on a daily basis. The downside of the transition into retirement is the problem of coming to the end of the day realizing you accomplished nothing of significance. When you accomplish little, you feel unfulfilled. Tracy's foundational focus poured into intentionally building and strengthening relationships. She labors joyfully now by forming new relationships.

Digging deeper into the lives of others reaps the opportunity to sow fruitful influence.

Quest

Have you deeply pondered what brings you great joy and value?

Do thoughts about retirement excite you or stir up dread?

What was the best day of your life? Why? What made it special?

Seed Thought

Tracy said, "If you prepare for retirement by identifying what matters most to you, then you multiply the chances of finding a continual purpose in life as the years go by."

Retirement brings more opportunities, time, and control. Also, the level of wisdom and understanding (based on the passage of time and our collection of experiences) should direct us to a deeper understanding of ourselves, the world, and other people allowing us to make significant, meaningful differences.

In the 1994 movie *The Shawshank Redemption*, Tim Robbins plays a banker named Andy Dufresne, who is sentenced to two life sentences in prison for murders he did not commit. Dufresne eventually escapes through a tunnel he laboriously dug over many years and takes with him the money he had been responsible for laundering for the crooked prison warden. At one point he says, "That's the way it is. It's down there and I'm in here. I guess it comes down to a simple choice, really. Get busy living or get busy dying."

If an intelligent and innocent banker can outsmart his jailers, so can you. Even if you are the jailer. Focus on what you have at hand and use it creatively. **The most valuable gift you have to offer anyone is yourself.** Finding the meaning and purpose for your life allows you to maximize the impact you can make on others and the joy you will experience on the journey. Don't wait — get busy living.

↗ **NOTE TO SELF**

It is not about how far you traveled,
but did you love the trip and significantly
share it with others?

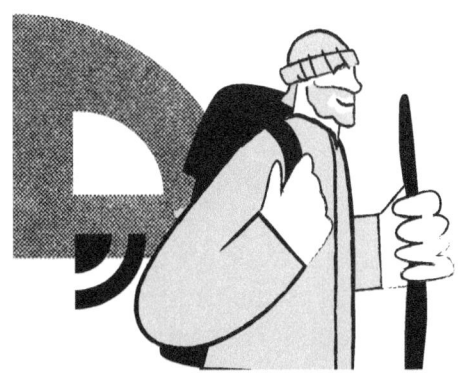

Michael the ROUTINEER

" *You are never too old to set a new goal or dream a new dream.* **"**

C.S. LEWIS

What will you miss if you only view retirement as an ending?

Focus

Deeply entrenched in the minds of many Americans is an independent and self-centered model of retirement. Beware of not needing other people. Retirement is not about the individual. Almost 400 years ago, John Donne wrote, "No man is an island, entire of itself; every man is a piece of the continent, a part of the main."

Other people matter, and our relationship to them matters, regardless of our age or status in life.

To find a fulfilling, energizing, and successful retirement, be flexible enough to overcome the programming we receive from society and culture. A self-focused notion of retirement sounds appealing until you live it. Many people achieve the "goal" only to discover emptiness. Change your thinking and set yourself on the path to significant retirement.

Michael's Journey

I sat down with Michael on a Saturday morning to talk about his life now two years into retirement following a successful career in the health care industry. I knew his secure financial status from our time working together for fifteen years preceding his retirement. I also perceived his high-level, driven personality. Our original work stemmed from his search for adjustment solutions in response to the massive growth of his company.

Five years before our first meeting, Michael started a small company with around twenty workers that had soared to more than 300 employees. The management style he used for the smaller version of the company did not work for the larger firm.

Michael described it this way: "You told me to stop looking at things as a problem. Instead, see them as a challenge. I thought you were playing word games. In fact, I went home the first night and told my wife what I thought about your word spinning. Fortunately, she knew better!"

I asked Michael a series of questions. At first, he reacted as if they were intrusive and annoying. But over time those questions helped him adapt his thinking to create a new model. By his own description, Michael's hands-on style with his team was the problem. His controlling detail in directing people made it "his" company rather than "theirs". He wanted his employees to take initiative and treat the work as if they were the owner. So, we talked about adapting and creating a different management model. Among the questions: What would help the company most? What would make it continue to grow and be healthy? How could we have many leaders rather than one?

Together we put a program in place to nurture team thinking and leadership skills. The business flourished as he transitioned from telling people what to do to encouraging them to take responsibility for finding ways to respond to challenges and move the company forward. It worked successfully, causing continued growth for the company.

Now two years into his retirement, we sat down, and before I could even start the conversation with my prepared questions,

Michael told me, "I am seriously thinking about living in Africa for a couple of years."

His statement shocked me. "Why would you choose such a major transition?" I asked.

"A higher purpose," he replied. "My two years of retirement have been awful. Not at all what I expected. I didn't realize how much I needed a challenge."

By all standards, Michael had it made. Healthy with no financial worries at all and resources to do anything he wanted, he told me, "I thought retirement was an ending. I looked forward to relief from work stress. I thought I would play golf whenever and wherever I wanted. I dreamed of taking a nap any time of day. I planned to watch a lot of sports on television and in person."

But when he followed that path, living the American retirement dream, he hated it. He worked hard for many years to enjoy the "easy life" in retirement, but the "easy life" left him feeling empty and worthless. Trapped in maintenance living gave him no purpose. Then everything changed. Knowing his expertise in the field, an old friend asked him to come to Kenya to help the government improve their health care system.

Michael said, "The trip to Kenya changed me. I saw a whole new world there like nothing I had ever seen. The extreme poverty and needs took me by surprise. But I didn't just see problems, I saw solutions in my head everywhere I looked. My energy level instantly shot through the roof! My wife says I came home acting like a kid again."

"Tell me more," I said.

"I am so thrilled," Michael replied. "I am going back to Kenya soon for a much longer visit. My skills and knowledge can make a difference for an entire nation!"

The challenges reinvigorated him. He had discovered his new purpose.

Before our meeting ended, Michael asked me, "Why didn't you tell me retirement requires adjustments?"

The truth is I had not considered it in those terms. He needed to repeat the process we went through to change his management style at his company, but this time directed toward his retirement life. His previous focus on building enough wealth to coast through retirement without any worries succeeded, but he found it unsatisfying. He now needed the flexibility to change and adapt to new plans.

Just as we restructured his business plan, Michael began restructuring his retirement model. He identified a new definition of success — not what he could get or keep, but what he could give. He put a new focus on the future to make a difference for others. For him, the emphasis of his giving moved from financial to the use of his experience and ability to help an entire nation.

 Michael's primary Retirement Mindset is Routineer.

 His secondary tendency is Seeker.

- He loves controlling detail.
- He has the heart of an inventor.
- The brain of a programmer.
- The attitude of an explorer.

His story is continually finding the next challenge in life.

What "good" challenge do you face in retirement?

Discoveries

Challenges Spur Growth

Strong trees do not grow in a greenhouse. They need the pressure of the wind to strengthen and develop their roots. In 1991 with the five-year construction of Biosphere 2 completed near Tucson, Arizona, the artificial environment for scientists to study living systems began. It soon provided us with new information. Scientists learned that while trees grow fast in an isolated environment, they do not fully develop and tend to fall over. Trees need wind, just as people need challenges. Allow the winds of challenge to bring purpose and joy to your retirement.

Michael moved from emptiness and a sense of worthlessness to joy and energy for life when he adapted his definitions and plans away from what many people think (and what he previously thought) would make for retirement success to doing what really mattered most to him. The return he got from putting his life into improving the medical system in Kenya cannot be measured on a balance sheet, but it is enormous. Without the flexibility to change his vision of retirement, he would have missed his purpose.

Money Really Isn't Everything

It is nice having enough money, but money alone is not enough. The choices permitted through resources are wonderful. But if you stop contributing to others, your bank balance may be large, but your life balance will be empty. Michael startled a friend one day by saying, "Can you believe it? I am bankrupt!"

"No way!" his friend said.

Michael explained, "Concerning money, I have plenty, but inside I feel bankrupt of meaning and purpose."

Life without meaning brings no satisfaction. Life wealth is more valuable than financial wealth.

Michael's wife said, "My husband is back again! He found joy and peace when he discovered a real challenge. Getting his focus off himself and onto others has reignited the enthusiasm of his spirit that made me originally fall in love with him."

Exercise the Power of Giving

Leisure, enjoyment, and relaxation are wonderful, but alone they lead to a sense of meaninglessness. The assumptions we make and the focus we choose can lead to a loss of purpose. Our investments in the lives of others provide a far more valuable and important return than any financial instrument can provide. Booker T. Washington said, "I think I began learning long ago that those who are happiest are those who do the most for others."

Being part of helping others develop a brighter future boosts your own mental, emotional, and even physical well-being. In fact, most people find they receive far more than they give when choosing this focus. Often the greater impact is made not through financial contributions, but through the gift of experience, skills, and time.

As the old saying goes, "Money is a wonderful servant, but a terrible master."

Craft a Life Mission Statement

Before making new policies and procedures for Michael's business, we crafted a mission statement serving as the guide for everything to follow. If it would help achieve the mission, we made the change, and if it would not, we passed. That became our road map. After our conversation, Michael formulated his life mission statement — **I live to leave this world a better place by helping others.**

Your mission statement should reflect your values and whatever matters most to you. The mission is not limited by what others expect. Your mission may not require great resources, and no one (except you) can hinder you from reaching and achieving your purpose. Enhance the value and meaning of your life by clearly defining your goals and purpose. Do so as early in life as possible. Make your mission big and meaningful enough to carry you with clarity of focus through your entire life!

Do What You Can

Centuries ago, the British statesman, Edmund Burke, said, "No one ever made a greater mistake than the man who did nothing because he could do only a little."

Aging naturally diminishes some level of our strength and health. But those who sit down and do nothing for long enough find they can no longer do much of anything. The greatest losses are suffered by those who let the limitations of what they can do stop them from doing anything.

Therefore, do not withdraw from life because you have experienced the loss of your once youthful strength and energy. The important thing is not to do everything, but to do something. Maybe you can only give two or three hours a week. Those may be the most important hours in someone's life. Maybe you can only invest in one person rather than many. Do what you can. Whether it is physical or mental, the principle is the same: The more we do, the more we will be able to do.

Quest

Did you leave your life mission behind when you left your working career?

How can you identify and make necessary adjustments to your retirement plan?

Have you given up because you cannot do all the things you once did?

Seed Thought

At the beginning of Michael's story, we quoted from John Donne's famous Meditation Seventeen. The year before publication in 1624, Donne nearly died. He lost two stillborn children. Then three other children died very young. When his beloved wife, Anne, died five days after giving birth to their last child, Donne entered a period of great depression.

His days of carefree travel and dangerous adventures ended. Instead, Donne took a position as a vicar in the Church of England and served as royal chaplain to King Charles I. He poured his heart into his sermons and poems, touching the lives of others.

By maintaining flexibility and adaptability, you not only improve your own life, but you also make a greater impact on others.

Donne's poem, "No Man is an Island", ends with these words: "Any man's death diminishes me, because I am involved in mankind, and therefore never send to know for whom the bell tolls; it tolls for thee."

> ↗ NOTE TO SELF
>
> Automatic transmission makes driving a car easier but in driving your life, knowing how and when to change gears and direction puts the fun of control back in your hands.

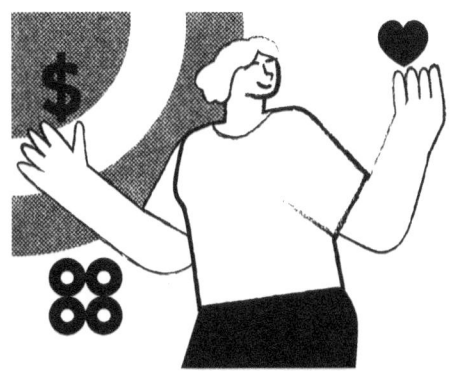

Gail the SEEKER

" *Financial resources enable, but do not determine, enjoyment of life in retirement.* "

ROBERT MORISON

Does perspective on money impact retirement success?

Focus

Not all dollars are equal. Obviously, from a standard accounting perspective, every dollar holds the same purchasing power. But mental accounting differs from standard accounting in that it adds or subtracts the psychological value attributed to dollars earned. For many, their work provides more than subsistence. For instance, it provides a sense of identity, belonging, accomplishment, and purpose — all potentially positive psychological benefits. If work provides a sense of self-actualization and personal growth, the psychological value of the income is even higher.

On the other hand, work may produce stress, frustration, and separation from family — all on the negative, or cost side of mental accounting. The total perceived value of the income from work is the total of economic value plus or minus the psychological benefits and costs. Not surprisingly, from a mental accounting perspective, equivalent retirement income seldom produces psychological benefits at the same level as work income.

This explains why a retiree whose standard accounting retirement income remains equivalent to work income sometimes feels important positive psychological elements of their life are now missing. Losing relationships with colleagues and work friends, not having an established avenue for making contributions to achieving goals, and not being recognized by colleagues and others for your contributions all create potentially major voids in your retirement life and can reduce your overall happiness as a retiree.

To get the mental accounting ledgers back in balance, or to even exceed the pre-retirement ledger balances, you must identify what is important in your mental accounting framework and develop a plan to bring more of it into your retirement life. An important part of that plan is understanding what drives your sense of happiness and well-being and the key mindsets and attitudes essential for developing those well-being drivers.

The key to this mindset is found in the work of Carol Dweck, who developed the notions of fixed and growth mindsets.[8] Individuals with a fixed mindset view themselves as having little or no ability to change who they are or will be. In other words, their mindset is "fixed" in terms of development, skill acquisition, and change in general. Growth mindsets see challenges as growth opportunities. For retirees who face replacing their drivers of life satisfaction, a growth mindset is critical. Retirement must be viewed as another productive phase of life with the potential to provide greater levels of well-being than any life phase preceding it.

Armed with self-knowledge, an understanding of well-being drivers, and a growth mindset, a potential retiree or already retired person is equipped to embark on a successful retirement. This success comes through offsetting the mental accounting deficits money income alone cannot measure.

Gail's Journey

I ran into Gail, a friend I had not seen in years, one evening at a benefit dinner for a

---

[8]   Dweck, C. (2006). *Mindset: The New Psychology of Success.* New York: Ballantine Books.

local not-for-profit organization. She asked if I would be willing to meet with her and her husband, Jerry, to discuss her recent retirement. So, we met for coffee at my office a few days later. After being seated around my small conference table, she said bluntly, "I am six months into my retirement, and it has fallen far below my expectations."

She continued, "I am embarrassed to confess, but I retired without giving retirement much thought or planning. Since I didn't have a plan, I don't understand why I feel so unfulfilled already."

"Tell me more," I said.

"It is not like I set specific goals and have some inability to reach them. It's more of a sense of emptiness," she replied.

Jerry joined the conversation saying, "I had planned to retire in about a year, but we decided I would continue working, *not because we need it*, but to provide an even better financial foundation. We both have pensions, 401ks, social security benefits, home equity, some other investments, and cash savings. We are in excellent financial shape. However, watching Gail has made me apprehensive about retirement."

"But," Gail said, "something is out of balance."

She continued, "I used to love receiving a paycheck because it reminded me of all the work I did with colleagues, customers, and by myself to earn that check. I felt I was a good partner and problem solver. I sensed great accomplishment and self-worth. The same feelings continued even when the company changed to payroll direct deposits. But now, money from investment accounts, pension checks, and social security checks fail to give me that good feeling. And I really miss it!"

"What do *you* think is at work here?" I asked.

"Maybe I was a workaholic and didn't know it," she replied.

"You do always like to stay busy," Jerry agreed.

Gail continued, "It seemed like the money I received for my work carried more satisfaction with it than the money I get from pensions and investments. I interacted with people and helped get things done providing a sense of accomplishment. Even though our team members didn't express appreciation to one another frequently, the regular checks seemed to convey their appreciation."

She paused for a moment and then said, "You asked what I think is causing this. I think my work checks lifted part of me and retirement checks do not. It's just money. Is this just crazy? Why do I perceive some money as different from other *money*?"

I sipped my coffee and thought about Gail's comments for a few moments. Then I asked, "Have you ever heard of Abraham Maslow?"

They both recognized the name, but nothing more.

I explained, "The psychologist Abraham Maslow wrote a paper in 1943 entitled 'The Theory of Human Motivation' in which he introduced his hierarchy of human needs."[9]

Jerry, kiddingly (I think), hinted that Maslow's Hierarchy is older than I am. After a good laugh, I drew a reasonable representation of Maslow's Hierarchy on a napkin and slid it over to them.

---

[9]   Maslow, A. (1943). "A Theory of Human Motivation, Psychological Review, 50(4), 370-396.

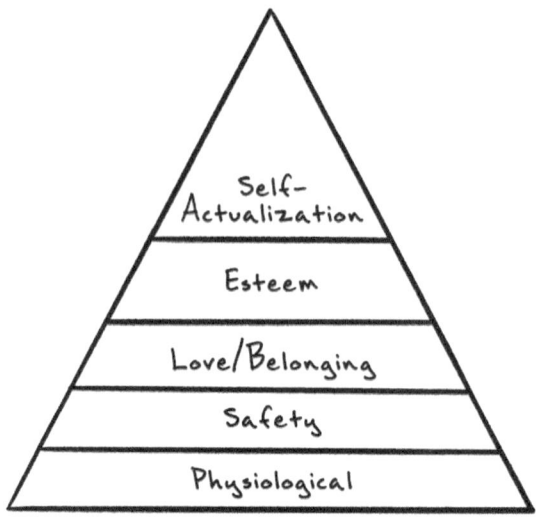

Maslow's Hierarchy of Needs

"Maslow's Hierarchy gives practical insights into how to think about your present situation. The bottom two levels of Maslow's Hierarchy relate to basic human needs. The very bottom level concentrates on food, water, clothing, shelter, staying warm — the necessities of life. If these basics are missing, people tend to focus on seeking them. The next level, security, focuses on personal safety and securing necessities over time. The third level focuses on the need to belong and to have meaningful relationships. The need for esteem from accomplishments is level four. The final level, self-actualization, involves reaching one's full potential — where you lead the life you were born to lead."

"Look at my drawing," I said. "How might this information apply to understanding your life back when working and now in retirement?"

The gears in Gail's mind began churning.

After a minute or so, she responded, "I think my payroll checks satisfied my physiological and security needs. And they also reflected my sense of belonging generated from contributing to successful work teams. So, I think my paychecks contributed to achieving perhaps all the first four levels of needs in Maslow's Hierarchy."

After deeper discussion we discovered some of her company's goals, especially sustainability, were consistent with her highest aspirations, meaning she was also satisfying self-actualization needs. So, her paychecks filled the needs and values on all levels of Maslow's Hierarchy.

Gail said, "My retirement income does not come with any sense of being valued by colleagues or pursuing higher goals or the subsequent sense of self-actualization. I am now missing the top two levels."

"Gail," I asked, "what are you doing now in retirement to replace the needs previously satisfied at work?"

"Well, I do some work with a local food bank and another not-for-profit group assisting veterans struggling with the emotional impacts of multiple deployments," she answered.

"And don't you get some sort of esteem and self-actualization from your volunteer work?" I asked.

"Yes. Their facial expressions and words of thanks do affirm me. I developed and implemented a better inventory system at the food bank. And I felt quite valued for it on receiving a round of applause at a recent food bank staff meeting."

At that moment, it dawned on Gail she was getting social connection and affirmation of value, *but now it had no connection to her paycheck.*

"Gail," I said. "Think about friends you connect with now in retirement. Think about your resurrected tennis skills and regular tennis matches with friends and Jerry, and your other family members who love seeing a less-stressed version of you on a regular basis. How do these relationships satisfy your needs for being cared about and loved?"

After a brief pause, she replied, "Okay, so the first four levels of Maslow's Hierarchy are currently being satisfied in my retirement but levels three and four come from something other than work and my paycheck. But, what about self-actualization? Where do I find more of that?"

"Keep looking. Continue the growth mindset you used throughout your working life. Your retirement is wide open with opportunities to grow. Begin to think about retirement being more valuable than a paycheck. Rekindle relationships that create acceptance and belonging. And seek out new opportunities to create value for a new set of people," I said.

I continued, "Let's give you some time to consider all we have talked about and meet again later to see if a lack of self-actualization is still on top of your mind. Is it possible you are already doing the very things capable of bringing you joy and self-actualization? We will continue this conversation whenever you decide you are ready."

As we closed, Jerry said, "I am so glad I tagged along for this meeting. It's opened my eyes to my own need to be planning so retirement will not hit me so abruptly!"

When we met three months later, Gail exclaimed, "Thank you! I have increased my volunteer work at the food bank, and I get a great sense of satisfaction and purpose from that work. Jerry has seriously begun work on planning his retirement transition. I am now very satisfied with my retirement!"

 Gail's primary Retirement Mindset is Seeker.

 Her secondary tendency is Planner.

- She loves making a difference in service.
- She has the brain of a business manager.
- The attitude of an achiever.

Her story is one of transferring meaning from a paycheck to relationships.

What brings you satisfaction that is not found in a paycheck?

Discoveries

Work Is More Than a Paycheck

Gail wrapped almost everything meaningful about her work into her paycheck. This is understandable as humans often try to convert things difficult to measure into things easier to measure. Using salary as a proxy is not necessarily a bad thing, but it can become an issue when the salary goes away and recognition of everything being measured by salary fades away with it.

Separation Theorem

Recognizing work as more than a paycheck brings valuable insight in Gail's story by showing which elements of work satisfied which needs in Maslow's Hierarchy of Needs. If everything gets bundled in your paycheck, revealing what moves you up and down the hierarchy becomes a challenge. When you know elements of your work can be "separated" and considered in isolation, it is easier to see the steps connected to your needs. It also makes the retirement transition easier since you separated financial and non-financial elements and can now work on each as you wish.

Needs Vary and Retirement is a Team Sport

You are unique and have unique needs. Your spouse or significant other is unique and has unique needs. Therefore, clearly approach mapping out retirement as a collaborative effort. Retirement income provides the opportunity to replace and reposition needs once filled by the workplace. In retirement, the opportunity is yours to design a new life satisfying your needs and the needs of those important to you. Certainly, these plans evolve over time, but active participation in the design process leads to self-actualization. The good news? You now own more control over your life than at any other time. The bad news? With control comes responsibility. If bad retirement days are the fault of a relentless boss, that boss is you. You are now in charge. Seize the day. Maintain healthy control of your life. If "control" is too strong a word for you, think of it in terms of shaping, influencing, and designing your own life.

Relationships Matter, Really

Studies indicate relationships are the basic elements of a successful retirement and longer life. Work is social in nature and many retirees point to the social interaction associated with work as one of the more enjoyable aspects of their work life. Developing relationships in retirement around shared goals or activities is critical in replacing relationships lost in transitioning to retirement. Working with not-for-profits and participating in various sports and activities with like-minded and goal-oriented people multiplies the creation of positive mental relationship benefits.

Quest

In retirement, what activities might you give up providing various levels of need satisfaction on Maslow's Hierarchy? And with what can you replace them with in retirement?

When you net out all the psychological benefits and costs of your work, what remains in your mental accounting balance?

When retired, how can you leverage your interests and skills to create value for others?

Which working relationships served as highly important to you and how can you develop new relationships providing similar benefits?

What activities move "self" aside allowing you to be completely absorbed in the moment? These may be the activities pointing the way to self-actualization in which you look back and say, "What a spectacular experience!"

Seed Thought

View the transitional changes of retirement in phases rather than as one abrupt change. By considering what needs your paycheck satisfies, you can begin to develop a transition plan to help you maintain or increase your sense of well-being in retirement. No "retirement-in-a-box" solution exists to make this go smoothly. Retirement is collaborative work requiring self-awareness and a growth mindset open to learning new things about yourself. The opportunity to design your life and pursue your own development arrives with amazing and unique possibilities. So, make retirement your ultimate adventure.

"Wealth is the ability to fully experience life." Henry David Thoreau

> ⟶ **NOTE TO SELF**
>
> It's not about the license or the car or the driving skill acquired through experience. Maybe it's not even the destination. Focus on the journey!

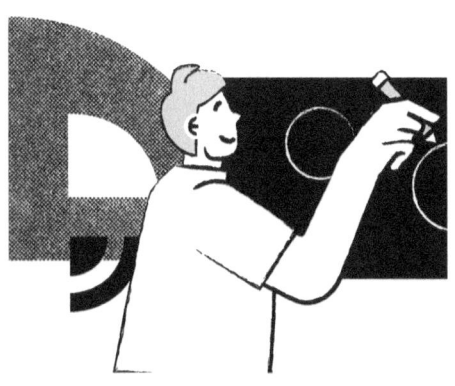

Ezra the ROUTINEER

" *An abundance of research strongly suggests that happiness, not just in later years but across the life span, is tied directly to the health and plentifulness of one's relationships.* **"**

ARTHUR C. BROOKS

Is what you think you are missing not the real problem?

Focus

People experience a sense of loss entering retirement. Many positives can be found in making this transition, but it is not uncommon for someone to wander around a few months or even years into their retirement suddenly encountering a strong sense something big is missing. Then they take steps to try to address the issue and fill the empty space. But many of those steps fail because the person taking them failed to identify the missing thing. So, no matter what they try, the void remains.

One benefit of retirement is the pause this transition gives you. **Take the opportunity to get in touch with what really motivates you and provides meaning in your life.** As we work with people in and nearing retirement, we find they struggle to identify things providing true meaning and satisfaction. But taking the time to look deeply on the inside pays huge dividends in life (even on the outside) because it allows you to focus your effort and energy on what matters most. We call this process "living inside out".

Ezra's Journey

Ezra embodies the mental picture of "a good guy". He is a loyal, hard worker. He is a smart man, a good thinker, and highly dependable. Ezra started working with a small trucking company right out of high school at the bottom of the ladder. His first job included washing and cleaning big rigs between their trips over the road.

After three months, Wayne, an older mechanic in the company, sat with Ezra at lunch. He noticed Ezra's positive character traits and the diligent way he worked. Wayne asked the owner of the company to let him train Ezra in his department. The growing company struggled at keeping up with more diesel engines running than their current staff could handle. He got permission to enlist Ezra as his helper.

Through the years Ezra's skill and knowledge grew. Ten years later, Ezra rose to become the top diesel mechanic in a fast-growing trucking company. Five years later, he managed a team of five other mechanics. They met impossible deadlines to keep the trucks on the road. Ezra and his team accomplished everything asked by the owner.

At the age of 68, Ezra retired from the trucking company. He had, for a long time, looked forward to retiring. But after a couple of years, he realized his zeal for meaningful living diminished. Ezra knew he needed help and invited me into a coaching discussion. In our first conversation, we did assessments to discover what he enjoyed in the past through his work at the trucking company.

"I think I actually miss the stress and the hectic pace of the company truck maintenance shop," said Ezra.

"So do you think operating your own small repair shop would bring some enthusiasm back in your life?" I asked.

"No. Not really. I have done some repair work for myself and a few friends. It didn't motivate me to want to keep doing it," he said.

"Could it be that something about your work other than the mechanical maintenance filled a sense of purpose for you?" I asked.

As we dug deeper into what he really valued in his work, Ezra said, "What I miss the most is helping other people do their job well. Wayne, my mentor, taught me all the things I needed for doing a good job as a mechanic for the company. When he left, the baton passed from him to me, and I started training the younger mechanics. I think this made me feel valuable."

"We call this an 'ah-ha' moment," I explained. "It's a moment of revelation suddenly bringing power to alter direction for everything yet to come. What do you think is your next step?"

"I am not sure," he answered.

"I suspect someone also followed your example when you left your work position, but you may be feeling like you still hold a 'baton' with great value and you struggle with what to do with it now," I said.

"I suggest you sit down with your wife and grown children. Ask them what they see in you that might bring potential value to others. Let others help you identify places you can invest your time and skills. I think your idea of 'passing the baton' may provide you direction for the satisfaction now missing in your retirement."

One of his daughters, a third-grade teacher, presented a brilliant idea to him. Two boys in her class desperately needed a strong male role model, which each lacked in their lives. They also needed to grow their skills, especially in reading.

"Please come to my class for an hour or two twice a week. You will be helping me, these two boys, and maybe even yourself," she pleaded.

Ezra told me later, "I would never have come up with this challenging idea on my own. In fact, I thought it might be a bad idea."

Nevertheless, he decided to give it a try. The results enormously changed his life.

Five years passed. The first boys Ezra helped moved up to junior high school. And Ezra still continues going to third grade twice a week. Each year new kids need help. Ezra invests in far more than just their reading skills. He models a successful and meaningful life for these young kids bringing his natural knack for finding their interests. Then he motivates them to face difficult challenges they believe are impossible.

For example, those first two boys loved sports more than anything. Ezra chose books for them to read focused on sports. One thing led to another, and soon Ezra found himself serving as the baseball and basketball coach for third graders at the school. After a couple of seasons, he was asked to train other volunteer coaches in how to relate to their players in ways beyond just teaching skills for the sport.

Ezra's new "career" didn't come with a job title or a paycheck.

But he says, "The benefits are amazing!"

Since he now "passes the baton" of skills through meaningful time in relationships, retirement no longer feels meaningless and boring. Zeal and excitement flow from knowing and pursuing his new purpose in life.

Retirement offers opportunities to get in touch with what motivates you. Identify your motivators, put them into step-by-step practice, and discover the wonder of transformational change. In their book The *Power of Moments*, Chip and Dan Heath wrote, "Actions produce more insights than insights produce action."[10]

I placed this chart on the table for Ezra to examine. "Where on this life cycle chart have you been in retirement? Where are you now?"

---

[10]   Heath, C. and Heath, D. (2017). *The Power of Moments*, New York: Simon & Schuster.

Life Cycle©

Transitioning

- Being Creative
- Positive
- Learning
- Networking
- Optimistic
- Sensing New Purpose

Theme: On the Road Again

Life is Great!

- Living my purpose
- Active
- Committed
- Optimistic
- Energized
- Giving

Theme: Wow

Inner Searching

- Inner Thinking
- Looking at Values
- Quiet
- Questing
- Searching
- Inward Exploring

Theme: Hide & Seek

Disenchanted

- Stuck
- Reactive
- Resistant
- Bored
- Devalued
- Sad

Theme: Life is Tough

After studying the chart for a few minutes, Ezra said, "When we started, I was definitely stuck in the disenchanted section. Working with you, I made progress by moving into the inner searching area. Now I find myself on the top of the circle bouncing back and forth from transitioning to life is great."

"Good," I said. "You realize life is never stuck on great. We all bounce back to the transitioning phase which in turn can lead us back to the 'Life is Great' quadrant."

 Ezra's primary Retirement Mindset is Routineer.

 His secondary tendency is Seeker.

- He loves to share life skills in training others.
- He has the brain of a mechanic.
- He has the heart of a gentleman.
- The attitude of a server.

His story is finding meaningful service in basic education.

What do you have to give away for impacting the lives of others?

Discoveries

Ezra's story highlights the vital importance of identifying what really matters to you and how you can focus on those things.

In your life journey, start with exploring where you best "fit in".

Finding your purpose and passion begins with taking an honest self-assessment. No one knows what is within you better than you do. What is it you really enjoy doing? What makes a day a success to you on the inside? What have you struggled with, and what do you find easy? Do the challenges you overcame in the past tend to be the same type or widely different? There are many questions you could ask, but the main thing is to focus your attention on what really matters.

After you finish the self-assessment, we encourage you to buck up the courage to ask those who know you well, family, or close friends, to share their opinions of you. Most people find this step uncovers hidden truth — those close to you see things you do not see about yourself. They may give you insights you would never find on your own. Our blind spots blindside all of us. As a result, for some this second step may be more revealing than the first.

Consider scanning this QR code for a link to a self-assessment to help you identify your needs and values.

Ignore Preconceived Limitations

We tend to limit ourselves. We observe the outside world and what it thinks and how it operates. Then we allow our perceptions to dictate what we believe we can and cannot do. Ezra had no formal education beyond high school. He earned no degree credentials or specialized training that people normally expect from educators. He spent his career working with his hands. But Ezra exerts more impact on educational enrichment than many of the trained teachers in his town.

Hopefully, Ezra's story stimulated you to examine your own needs and values. It is vital for you to get in touch with your core values. You need to continue to find value in the use of your time and abilities to maintain your passion for life. If you do not first identify what brings you satisfaction, you will find yourself failing to find focus in the right direction. You may discover your purpose in something completely different from how you spent your career, or it may be a continuation of something once related to your job. The important thing is to not let yourself be limited by what you *think* rather than by what is *real*.

A Crucial Part of Looking Inside

Life is a spiritual journey. Some people react negatively to that statement because of their experiences with organized religion. But this is not about churches or religious groups, although for many people religion plays an important part of their lives as well as a source of meaning and purpose. What we are talking about is your inner being — the part that makes you who you really are. It is not height, weight, or any other characteristic outwardly defining us, but rather what we are on the inside. Most of us learn early in life to conceal our thoughts and feelings because of reactions from those around us. We learn that others often do not really want to know. In time, we learn to conceal things from even ourselves. An honest assessment of the realm inside us is fundamental for progress and growth.

Quest

How would those who know you best describe your passions and interests?

What are you doing in the present leading to real satisfaction and enjoyment?

How transparent are you able to be with people around you?

Seed Thought

The average person retiring at age 65 now lives over 18 years on average. Did you save the best for last? Do you want to go out in a blaze of glory? Would you settle for a simple glow of contentment?

It can be daunting and maybe terrifying to look deep inside. Some things we may prefer not to think about or remember. But the more open and honest we become with ourselves and with others, the less opportunities arise for our blind spots to deceive us. Things out in the open may cause pain, but pain reveals what needs to be healed. Dealing with repairs is the point of identifying and solving problems. Mysteries require a search. We all know life is not easy and all stages of life bring the refining fires. Search within. In other words, be honest with yourself. Let mentors, retirement coaches, friends, and family members help you bring the mystery within you out in the open for engaging your best possible expression of purpose and joy.

Jesse Owens said it well, **"The battles that count aren't the ones for gold medals. The struggles within yourself — the invisible, inevitable battles inside us all — that's where it's at."**

→ ## NOTE TO SELF

Don't travel alone. Know yourself. Learn your blind spots. And remember the back seat driver's irritating correction just might save your life.

Moving Forward

Retirement should be the dream chapter of your life, but a satisfying and meaningful retirement is not automatic. A retirement generating wonderful memories requires attention, thinking, planning, and effort on your part. It isn't like a fully guided two-week tour of Europe where everything is planned and executed by others, nor is it like a two-week unstructured vacation where whatever happens, happens. Your retirement likely will last two decades or longer. It may provide you with more time to utilize as you choose than ever before. This time and control mean you get to decide what is most meaningful to you and how to proceed in pursuing your dreams.

This book helps position you to take the action necessary to create your unique "Dream Chapter" of retirement. You have learned about the four primary retirement mindsets, the power of questions through the "Four Big Questions" of life and a collection of other very important questions to help you understand yourself, and the stories of real people struggling with retirement challenges and opportunities.

The Four Big Questions

Questions are the foundation of this book. Throughout the book, developing answers to The Four Big Questions in life motivate growth and discovery. These four questions are:

- **Who am I with my strengths?**
- **Where do I fit in?**
- **Who cares?**
- **What are my choices and who decides?**

While important throughout one's life, these questions can become even more important as you contemplate or experience retirement because the answers before and after retirement can change drastically. Just like exams in school, the questions seldom change, but the answers do. Anticipating the changes in your answers to these questions is at the heart of a successful transition from career to retirement.

Other important questions in each episode contribute to answering the Big Questions and are designed to help you make sense of who you are and who you want to become in retirement. Your retirement is unique to you, and you alone, so every individual reading this book will have different answers to the questions — and they are all correct answers! Who you are and what is meaningful to you is up to you.

One thing, however, is certain: the more time and effort you put into answering the questions throughout the book, the greater the benefits will be. The questions throughout the book can be quickly answered off the top of your head, but the more you work to get beyond the first and obvious responses, the more you will benefit. Some of the questions may stump you, while other questions may benefit from input from others who know you well and whose judgment you trust to assess the extent to which you're thinking about who you are aligns with theirs. Diligence and effort are your friends in your journey to discover your authentic self. So, you may want to go through the book and reconsider your initial answers to some or all the questions as you work to find your authentic self.

The Power of Stories

This book is built on real life stories gleaned from coaching people on retirement. Some of the stories reflect planning for retirement and other issues experienced in retirement. These stories are intended to be examples of specific problems and opportunities experienced by real people. While these stories by no means explore all possible retirement scenarios, they illustrate the essential nature of the issues and opportunities facing you as you plan and live in retirement. Your actual issues and opportunities may vary in type and intensity, but the narratives provide evidence of a path forward. The stories also encourage you to think of your life's story and how you can shape it. You are not alone in planning and living the Dream Chapter of your life.

Retirement Is a Team Activity

If you have a significant other, retirement planning becomes more complicated. If you and your significant other both work, retirement timing can become an issue as numerous factors may affect each of your retirement decisions. If your goal is to travel or move to another city and your spouse does not want to retire for five more years, then your retirement decision may be affected, or vice versa. Even if only one of you is working, retirement merits conversations with your significant other to ensure expectations, needs, and wants are coordinated. So, retirement conversations with your significant other are a must.

It may be helpful if your significant other takes our Retirement Mindsets Survey reads this book, and explores his/her own thinking by working through its questions. Comparing answers to the questions in this book may provide an excellent starting point for conversations and facilitate a better understanding of one another now and in retirement. Developing a clearer understanding of retirement mindsets and your own thinking puts you in a better position to have meaningful conversations with your significant other.

Another Resource: Our Dream Chapter Retirement Guidebook

Our work with clients revealed the value of good tools in planning and executing meaningful retirements. We have successfully used the materials in this book with clients for years and it has provided them with an excellent approach to thinking about the issues in retirement. In addition, we have developed and used a significant number of other practical tools with our clients. We share the best of these tools in our new *Retirement Guidebook*. To assist you to understand specific areas needing attention in your retirement planning, the *Guidebook* comes with access to our proprietary Retirement Awareness Survey. The *Guidebook* contains hands-on, practical, action-oriented tools to help you answer Retirement's Big Questions.

Meet the Authors

Charlie Baker,
Co-founder of Dream Chapter™
and Co-Founder of the CC Group
(Comprehensive Coaching)

Who is Charlie Baker? For over 30 years, Charlie's executive coaching experience spanned multiple industries. From higher education, retail industry, regional health care providers, energy clients, governmental agencies, and an international professional service corporation, he has consulted with those in the corporate suites and throughout the organizations to create and implement healthy, dynamic plans of action. His background of a B.S. in Education and a Master's in Theology laid the foundation for his passion of creating a workplace environment conducive for businesses to succeed and for their leadership at all levels to grow, thrive, and serve.

When not traveling, one can find him training for 5K's, working on the ranch, or spending quality time with his family.

During the latter years of his career, he 'dreamed' of helping others transition from their full-time, professional careers to their active, meaningful retirement years. What you hold in your hands is the fulfillment of that 'Dream Chapter'.

Larry Wofford, Co-founder of Dream Chapter™

Larry Wofford is a professor of innovation and entrepreneurship. As an entrepreneur, he developed and operated successful businesses in the logistics and motor vehicle industries. He, also, served on numerous boards, including the board of a national health-care organization. In his academic career, he has published two textbooks and numerous research articles.

Larry earned a Ph.D. in finance and real estate at the University of Texas at Austin and a Postgraduate Diploma from the University of Oxford. He is an urban planner, holding the AICP designation from the American Institute of Certified Planners. Larry is a Fellow of the Royal Institution of Chartered Surveyors and a Hoyt Fellow of the Homer Hoyt Advanced Studies Institute.

He has coached and guided many individuals making life and career decisions and transitions. It became his mission to develop an approach to help human beings experience meaningful and satisfying lives in retirement.

Craig Bothwell,
Co-founder of Dream Chapter™

Craig Bothwell spent 43 years as a successful executive and entrepreneur in the hospitality industry. What began as a college job washing dishes in 1969 with Mazzio's

Corporation, Craig found his passion for business and played a major role the next 36 years nurturing and rapidly growing the regional pizza chain and its subsidiary brands to over 200 locations and 3,000 employees. He served as President and Chief Operating Officer from 1986-2005.

In 2005, Craig left Mazzio's to become a franchisee for McAlister's Deli. He expanded to twenty restaurants in the Midwest before selling the company in 2012. Craig is also past president of the Oklahoma Restaurant Association (ORA) and continues to serve as an Associate Board Member. He is a partner and co-founder of The CC Group, a comprehensive coaching firm for business professionals eager to sustain success in life, work, and retirement through a proven and unique coaching process.

A native of Springfield, Missouri, Craig holds a Bachelor of Science degree in psychology from the University of Tulsa.